Veterinarian's Treasury

of

Practice Tips

Submit practice tips to:

Seymour Glasofer, D.V.M.
Newport News Animal Hospital
4504 Jefferson Avenue
Newport News, Virginia 23607

Lester Mandelker, D.V.M.
1631 West Bay Drive
Largo, Florida 33540

VETERINARIAN'S TREASURY OF PRACTICE TIPS

Compiled by: Seymour Glasofer, D.V.M.
Lester Mandelker, D.V.M.

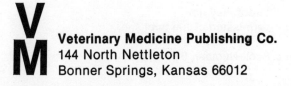

Veterinary Medicine Publishing Co.
144 North Nettleton
Bonner Springs, Kansas 66012

"A veterinarian should strive continually to improve his veterinary knowledge and skill, making available to his colleagues the benefit of his professional attainments, and seeking, through consultation, assistance of others when it appears that the quality of veterinary service may be enhanced thereby." (Section IV, A.V.M.A. *Principles of Veterinary Medical Ethics*)

This book is dedicated to our colleagues who have contributed many of these ideas.

Table of Contents

Preface   1

Introduction   3

Chapter   1.   General Management   5

Chapter   2.   Office Management   11

Chapter   3.   Client Relations   15

Chapter   4.   Employee Relations   24

Chapter   5.   Radiology   30

Chapter   6.   Laboratory   35

Chapter   7.   Pharmacy   40

Chapter   8.   Anesthesia   45

Chapter   9.   Surgery   51

Chapter   10.   Medical   67

Chapter   11.   Treatment   80

Contributors Index   125

PREFACE

The purpose of this book is to provide, in one source, practical ideas for the veterinary practitioner. It has been written and accumulated by practitioners solely for the benefit of practitioners. It is not a detailed complex medical textbook. Instead, it is a concise source of ideas from hundreds of veterinarians experiencing day to day problems.

Use of material that has previously appeared in Veterinary Medicine/Small Animal Clinician "Practice Pointers" and "That's A Good Idea" is acknowledged and appreciation is extended to the publisher and editor for permission to use this material.

The authors gratefully acknowledge the large number of veterinary practitioners, instructors, technicians, supplier's representatives, pharmaceutical companies, physicians, extension service staffs, etc., whose thoughts and suggestions are included. In some instances, a credit is not given for particular pointers because either the contributor requested anonymity or the source was inadvertantly lost.

Not every pointer or suggestion that appears here could be tested by the authors and no responsibility is assumed for any untoward reaction as a result of any procedure or technique. Retension of these pointers and practice tips can be improved by the study or consideration of only a limited number at one time. It is hoped that yearly additions and updating of these ideas and pointers can be accomplished. Any reader who has an idea or a better method is invited to contact the authors and share it with his colleagues.

By sharing these pointers and ideas, we will all benefit.

INTRODUCTION

A practice pointer or practice tip is a remedy to a practice problem that taxes your medical knowledge, ingenuity, and common sense. They usually fall somewhere between medical imagination and scientific fact. Practice tips simply apply successful solutions to common medical or business problems. They are often brief answers to complex situations. Rational thinking people devise practice tips. They are often nonconformists who aren't satisfied with customary medical ambiguity.

The practice tips philosophy simply involves finding the most successful solution to your practice problems and a willingness to share your solutions with colleagues. Some of our forefathers who utilized the practice tip philosophy made a lasting impression on the profession. They have given not only ideas but the more important motivation to "find a better way". Such contributions have been made by: John Bardens, Charlie Bild, George Burch, William F. Jackson, Robert Kirk, Harry Magrane, William Magrane, Jacob Mosier, James Yarborough . . . to name a few. Practitioners are best qualified to propose practice tips. Academicians can often give us the "best" solutions but many times sacrifice expedience and practicality. Researchers can give the knowledge and thoughts but the practitioner must implement them. What works well in the laboratory or under "ideal conditions", may not perform well in daily clinical applications. Many factors come into play for the practicing veterinarian. Only the practitioner can determine what is practical for him.

To develop the practice tip philosophy you must be a rational, well adjusted individual. There are no special powers required . You must be in the frame of mind to receive and comprehend knowledge. Your mind must not be cluttered with life's problems to the extent that you cannot adequately receive knowledge.

The authors urge you to set aside time to read, study and relax. "Escape" from problems and worries . . . through sports, movies, television, books or other recreational sources. "Study" your veterinary journals but also read other sources.

The more you read, the more sources you have to compare. Magazines, medical journals, folk and health medicine books, newspapers, etc., all may contain scientific material useful to you. Cut out articles and jot information down for later use. "Work off anger" in an acceptable way . . . take a long walk, run or exercise in any way. Schedule your life, not rigidly, but in such a way that each day includes time for rest, play, work, meditation and biological necessities. Take one thing at a time . . . try to solve each problem on its own without being obsessed about the next one coming.

Your profession, the practice of veterinary medicine, should turn you on and you must accept patient illness as a challenge and not give up easily. Know your limitations and seek help when necessary but you should not punish yourself for "failures". Remember, we are only human! Develop a plan to improve your input and frame of mind. Broaden your base, let your world grow larger. The more you experience, the more experiences you have. See what's new in the practice of medicine. Call a physician or local university on a complicated case. They generally love the challenge. Diagnose . . . Diagnose . . . Diagnose!!! This is the most consistent way to improve your knowledge base. Do work-ups and eliminate possible differential diagnoses by testing. Even if you can't immediately diagnose a problem completely by testing, at least you can tell what it isn't. This often is very helpful!

Relate to other rational well adjusted individuals. Relate to other colleagues and share problems and offer ideas. Think positive . . . think of a plan to improve continually. Think of practice pointers and develop the practice tip philosophy.

Lester Mandelker, DVM
Seymour Glasofer, DVM

Chapter/1

MANAGEMENT

It is a fact of life that a veterinarian's professional knowledge is not the sole determining factor of success or earning capability. If a practitioner is not aware of drug, equipment and procedural costs, if he has no check on employe integrity and ability, if the waste of supplies and time is allowed, the result can be business failure.

A legible and adequate record system is necessary to avoid getting lost in a sea of minutiae. This must document all monies received (if desired, a breakdown of amounts for different services) and an accounting for every dollar spent. Some form of inventory control is desirable, especially of items dispensed. Full details of all salaries, taxes withheld, deposited, etc., are mandatory. For the man or woman just entering practice, or for the practitioner wishing to update his record-keeping, various new systems are exhibited at national and some state meetings.

In any business, organization and efficiency are the rudiments of sound management practices but, we ultimately deal with individuals on a day to day basis. Our relationships determine our place in this world. The following management tips have been shared with you by people, veterinarians and businessmen alike, who have a good working knowledge and understanding of how to deal with people. We hope some of these ideas can be of benefit to you!

GENERAL MANAGEMENT TIPS

1. **PRICE ACCORDING TO QUALITY:** Most of us do not know or have forgotten that the priceless factor in a business operation is the love that goes into its making. This priceless factor cannot be purchased with money or any other material commodity. It is born of contented workers, well paid, respected, and appreciated, who are convinced their work is worthwhile and that they are rendering a service to humanity. The priceless factor, being love, cannot be put into a product unless there is love from the owner or boss down to the worker. With such a product, the purchase price becomes secondary, for its quality is so outstanding that it stands alone.

*** *** ***

2. **HUMAN RELATIONS DICTATE SUCCESS:** It is important to realize that when a veterinary practice is properly managed, the clients of the practice are satisfied and appreciative. The veterinarian is satisfactorily compensated, and the overall quality of the practice is high. Adequate human relations are the cornerstone of the properly managed veterinary practice. Unless the doctor has an understanding of the basic principles of human relations, either learned formally or gained instinctively, and applies them in managing his practice, his practice will fail because of client and personal dissatisfaction, plus failure to gain a sense of accomplishment. Application of proper human relations dictates whether a business is a success or failure. Failure is your inability to reach your goals in business, whatever they may be. The easiest way for you and your employees to improve your human relations is to take the Dale Carnegie human relations course.

*** *** ***

3. **WHAT IS YOUR PERSONALITY?** Don't be afraid to let it show. Be yourself. Don't copy others. You will attract others who like your personality and you will repel those who do not like your personality. Let the world see you as you are — your hobbies, your family, your professional interests. Remember, people who don't like your personality won't like your diagnosis, treatment, or fees. This is the basic rule of doing business. Think back — how many times have you really ever satisfied anyone who didn't like you?

*** *** ***

4. **CLIENT CONFIDENCE ESSENTIAL:** A veterinary practice is built on a satisfied clientele. You should be warmly and deeply client oriented. You must be sincerely interested in each client as a person, as well as being interested in their pet. You must display your expertise

6

and practice your art with complete assurance. This builds the client's confidence in you! For this reason, there are at least two times when veterinarian-client contacts are important; upon admission and upon discharge of the animal. Too frequently, the veterinarian allows his employees to receive and discharge patients. Such practice may result in a frustrated client with unanswered questions concerning his pet. A brief discussion with the client at the time of discharge will allow the veterinarian to talk about the pet's ailments, treatment received at the hospital, future care (including medication, husbandry, and diet). Often, the client is more concerned with the diet than the veterinarian is. The time of discharge is an excellent opportunity for a frank discussion of fees, which should have been discussed at the time the animal was admitted. Clear communications can save much time and prevent embarrassment. Be sure to give specific instructions on post-treatment care so the owner doesn't have to make a decision. Instruct exactly when you want to give another injection! Be positive and definite; not vague and unsure!!

******

5. THE FOUR JUDGEMENTS:
   A. How we look.
   B. What we do.
   C. What we say.
   D. How we say it.

******

6. SERVICE: The ability to empathize with your client and his animal's needs. Doing politely and kindly what the client wants.
Common service weaknesses:
   A. Telephone constantly busy.
   B. People waiting on the telephone line.
   C. Poor parking.
   D. Unpleasant, inadequate waiting room with offensive odors.
   E. Lack of warm greeting by office personnel.
   F. Clients required to wait too long.

******

7. BEWARE OF SUCCESS: Success is usually coupled with increased authority, and authority over others is always dangerous. When success is not accompanied with understanding, it is highly dangerous. When success is not coupled with true humility, it is explosive. The more authority we have, the greater the danger.

7

8. **THE MANAGERS CHIEF BUSINESS:**
   A. Organize the work to be done.
   B. Deputize who is to do the work.
   C. Supervise who does the work.

******

9. **KNOW YOUR COLLEAGUES:** Here's an easy way to know your colleagues better. Establish a regular, informal weekly luncheon in your area. Notify all practitioners who work in the area that a weekly luncheon will be held at a certain cafeteria or restaurant at the same time and day of each week. No reservations, no programs; just a chance to visit and have a good time. Doesn't make any difference if there's 2 or 20 present. People get to know each other better in a social environment.

******

10. **PRACTICE NEW TECHNIQUES:** Continuing education courses enlarge scientific knowledge. We go home with much new knowledge and good intentions. Like an Arab educated in the U.S.A., we can't apply learned techniques when we return to the home environment. When we return to our business, we don't apply new knowledge and equipment in our old, established, routine (rat race). We continue to maintain *"status quo"*.

    We need some way to help us change our routine — to get us out of our rut. Unfortunately, the only way we can change is by repeated application of the new knowledge or technique. Practice a new anesthetic technique; practice a new laboratory technique; practice being friendly; practice visiting a colleague; practice spending time with the family. Knowledge plus proper attitude often fails because one does not practice the activity. The law of learning is to do something frequently and regularly.

******

11. **SCHEDULE YOURSELF BUSY:** If you are just starting practice and have only a few appointments, schedule them close together — appear to be busy and in high demand without making people wait an inordinate length of time.

******

12. **GREET CLIENTS CHEERFULLY:** A happy client is the only advertising you need.

******

13. **RELAX:** You can conduct most of your clinical examinations while sit-

8

ting if you purchase an adjustable professional stool from a medical supplier. You will be less fatigued and more relaxed in your dealings with clients.

******

14. **FOLLOW UP TREATMENT:** Make it a policy to schedule a post-treatment visit for a pet. The usual "give me a call in a few days if your dog isn't doing O.K," may be a disservice to yourself and to the client and his pet.

******

15. **CHECKLIST OF ELECTIVE SURGERY:** Recommending elective surgery is both good business and highly ethical. Veterinarians should have on hand a check list of elective surgery that will help people enjoy their pets to a greater degree. Claw removal, soft palate resection, external nose correction, tonsillectomy, castration and hysterectomy of old or middle-age animals all provide a beneficial service to the pet owner.

******

16. **AT THIS TIME:** When preparing a certificate regarding an animal's health status, use the words "at this time" to help avoid misunderstanding if there should be a change in the animal's condition at a later date.

******

17. **TAPE INSTRUCTIONS TO CAGE:** Write special instructions for caged patients (*e.g.* feeding directions, fecal check wanted, etc.) on labeling or masking tape and apply over the door latch. The tape sticks easily and cannot be overlooked.

******

18. **USE FATIGUE MAT:** If you have terrazzo or tile floors, place a fatigue mat next to your operating table and examination table. You'll notice a big improvement in how your legs and back feel at the end of a busy day.

******

19. **RETURN ALL COLLARS, LEASHES, ETC. TO THE CLIENT WHEN A PATIENT IS ADMITTED:** If a rug, towel, or toy must be left to make the animal "feel at home", describe the object on the patient's record card so that no time is wasted in looking for it when the patient is discharged.

******

20. **SPECIAL TREATMENT TAGS:** To be certain that special instructions

are emphasized when an animal is admitted to the hospital, mount a peg board (2 ft × 4 ft) near the receptionist's desk. Hang tags of different colors on hooks that specify special treatment required (diet, urinalysis, immediate bathing, etc.). The tags are applied to, or accompany, the animal when it is taken to the kennel.

* * * * * *

21. **LOCATE CHALKBOARD IN WARDS:** An excellent way to call attention to special instructions in the hospital ward is to write them on a large chalkboard mounted in a prominent position in the ward.

* * * * * *

22. **ANNUAL PHYSICAL:** Develop a standard physical examination program for dogs over five years of age. Send the owners a reminder card for their pet's annual physical. Dogs should be examined twice a year after the age of eight. Laboratory examinations running from $7.00 to $10.00 including blood, urine and fecal, plus a $10.00 x-ray examination of the chest, and a $5.00 physical examination fee would make the annual physical run approximately $22.00 to $25.00.

* * * * * *

23. **DENTAL RECALL:** Prepare a reminder card for use in dental work. Dogs should be brought in once or twice a year for dental attention. Those dogs which have a real tartar problem may require more attention than this.

* * * * * *

24. **DEFINE EMERGENCIES:** Don't automatically accept a client's description of an emergency. It is perfectly ethical, and has a calming effect to say, "Please tell me the symptoms and we will decide if you have an emergency".

Chapter/2

OFFICE MANAGEMENT

As practitioners, we tend to think first of increasing efficiency in examination and surgery. However, increasing the efficiency of our office and clerical employees will also bear fruit. These members of the hospital staff will be more dedicated if they know their ideas are welcomed and will be considered. Let them be aware that their suggestions for saving time, money or effort are appreciated.

Your front office is a hub of important people and business transactions. Efficiency, pleasant attitudes, and consideration are primary concerns when dealing with the public. Here are some practice tips and ideas about office procedures.

OFFICE TIPS

25. **SIGN IN BOOK AIDS SERVICE:** For those not using an appointment system, have you thought about having a "sign in" book at the receptionist's desk so that each person entering the hospital will sign the book. A spiral notebook works well for this purpose. The following information is recorded:

    A. Name of the person.
    B. Whether or not they have been in the hospital before.
    C. The animal's name and complaint.

Post a sign, 'Please sign this book". This will give you a permanent record of the traffic flow in the hospital. It also is a good means for the receptionist to know who is next for professional attention. It will also help with client name recall. "The book" can make a hospital function more smoothly and help the receptionist immeasurably. Be sure your receptionist remembers that, to the client, their name is the most important sound — in any language. This registration procedure allows everyone to greet a client by name without having to ask.

******

26. **REDUCE CONGESTION IN RECEPTION ROOM:** If you do not practice on an appointment basis, have your receptionist suggest to clients that they call before they come in. The receptionist can then tell them at what time you are most likely to see them promptly.

******

27. **CONTROL THE TELEPHONE:** The telephone is a device with exceedingly "bad manners". It doesn't care whether you're tired, asleep, busy, happy, or unhappy. It will aggravate you and destroy your relationship with clients if you'll let it. For this reason, it is important that you make the telephone your servant. Develop a system that does not allow it to interfere with your work. No calls or interuptions while you're with a client. Return all calls at a regular time each day. If you find yourself being disagreeable and nasty on the phone, put up a mirror so that you will look at yourself while talking on the phone. You'll find you talk "nicer" when you look at your face during the conversation. If your telephone is upsetting your business and personal life, ask the phone company personnel for advice.

******

27. **GOODWILL BOOSTER:** If you anticipate being away from your practice and you take patients on a nonappointment basis, keep your clients from making a needless trip to the office by advising them to phone before their next visit. This simple display of thoughtfulness

toward clients is an excellent goodwill booster.

******

29. **MINIMIZE NO SHOW'S:** Have your aide call the client the day before an animal is scheduled for elective surgery. The call serves as a reminder of the appointment and provides an opportunity to repeat preoperative feeding instructions. This simple procedure minimizes the number of no-shows and gives you better utilization of your operating room time.

******

30. **QUIET PLEASE:** To minimize the ringing and buzzing noises common to most veterinary offices, replace bells and buzzers (telephone, door sentry, intercom system) with a chime or light signal, or both.

******

31. **BASIC CREDIT CONTROL:** When making out a record card for a new client, don't forget to make a note of the client's place of employment. Few clients object to giving this information and it is a great help when credit must be extended.

******

32. **A TACTFUL APPROACH TO CASH-ONLY PRACTICE:** To reduce the number of clients who request credit, place a small sign on the receptionist's desk reading "Payment required when services are rendered.".

******

33. **DRUG REACTION ALERT:** To save time, and as an extra precautionary measure, use file cards of a distinctive color for animals that have shown a reaction to any medication.

******

34. **ATTACH SNAP HOOKS ON CLIENT SIDE OF RECEPTIONIST'S COUNTER:** A dog's leash can be attached to these hooks while the owner is paying the bill or transacting other business with the receptionist.

******

35. **INCREASE SEATING CAPACITY:** For those occasions when entire families seem to accompany a pet to the office, keep a few folding chairs available (but out of sight).

******

36. **INTIMIDATED PATIENTS:** If a cat in the reception room is in-

13

timidated by dogs, put it into a cage elsewhere on the premises until it can be moved to an examining room.

******

37. **EASE ANIMAL TENSION:** When patients are brought into the office for a visit, offer them a pet vitamin. Most dogs and cats readily accept the vitamins and the gesture usually eases the animal's tension in the office. Some pets even begin to look forward to a return visit.

******

38. **INFORMATION CARD HELPFUL:** To save yourself and your receptionist much time, why not have each new client fill out a general information card when bringing a patient to the hospital? This small card can be used before the clinic card is made out.

Chapter/3

CLIENT RELATIONS

How do your clients describe you? Is their comment, "He repaired my dog's leg all right, but what a grouch"! Sometimes an in-depth analysis of every client contact is necessary. Include the way the receptionist and the doctor answer the phone, the greeting to the client when he enters the waiting roon, the veterinarian's demeanor in the examination room, his questioning about the request for payment for the services rendered. All of these situations can evoke a positive or a negative response from the pet owner.

A tape recording could be made in the examination room and studied. A common failing is that we take too much for granted. Consider the following: Is the client addressed by name? Is compassion shown for the pet or is the pet regarded as an object on the table? Do you say "Thank You"?

What is the best response when a client feels the fee is too high? Does the practitioner confronting the client remember "A soft answer turneth away wrath" and carefully explain the charges involved? Sometimes a further elaboration of just what has been done for the patient and a quiet reference to the fact that expenses are caught in an inflationary spiral will suffice. Sometimes a billing mistake is made and an apology is in order.

If clients leave your clinic angry or disgruntled, they are not apt to return for your services despite your professional skill. The following client relation tips will suggest some thoughts about how the client may visualize us. Hopefully, we can increase our understanding of human relations and improve our client relations.

CLIENT RELATIONS

39. **POSITIVE REINFORCEMENT:** Thank clients who are prompt for appointments and you will give them a reason to be on time in the future. Clients like doctors who say "Thank You".
Positive reinforcement creates the right kind of response between you and the other person. You could even say that it pays the other person, in advance, for doing something you want done.

******

40. **CLIENT CLASSIFICATION SYSTEM:** We need continually to re-emphasize the client classification technique if we're going to be truly happy in business. We all wish we could please and satisfy all clients, but this is absolutely impossible. Therefore, we should classify each client into one of four categories.
The "A" clients are completely "sold" on you. They tell everyone who will listen how great you are. You are happy with them, and they are happy with you.
The "B" clients are those people who also think you are great and believe wholeheartedly in you, but they do not "broadcast" their strong feelings about you (they are the silent type). You enjoy working with them, and they enjoy coming to you.
The "C" clients are those who are not particularly sold on you. They use your services because you are convenient, but are not loyal to you. You work for them without any real enthusiasm.
The "D" clients are the complainers, the criticizers, the price buyers. These people may not even like you. They don't trust you. They don't believe in you. Working for these people, generally, is unrewarding and often a terrible headache.
The obvious benefit in the A, B, C, D client system is that the more time we spend with our A and B clients (friends), the happier and the more rewarding our work is to us. So don't knock it until you've tried it. Mark each client's record card as follows: A = gold, B = silver, C = blue, D = red. Be sure all your employees give the A and B clients the V.I.P. treatment!!!

******

41. **VETERINARY HISTORY HELPFUL:** In addition to the usual information you obtain from clients on their first visit, it is also useful to learn (1) what their past experience with veterinarians has been; (2) who referred them to you; and (3) how psychologically important their pets are to them.

******

16

42. **AVOID NEGATIVE:** Good client relations require continual effort. If your hospital operates on an appointment system, be sure that any signs posted regarding appointments do not contain the word *only*. The sign should read, "Patients are received by appointment". Do not use *by appointment only*. This is poor (negative) public relations.

* * * * * *

43. **SPECIALIZATION HAZARDS:** One of the inherent dangers of specialization in any field is the lack of wholeness (limited interests and activities). Specialization may make for increased efficiency, but it leads to dehumanization. A lack of interest is the mark of the production line—cold, impersonal, reserved, unconcerned. The veterinarian who specializes must be aware of this danger. He can become so involved in his specialty that he forgets that people are involved. By all means, excel in some phase of veterinary medicine, but don't forget the human relations aspect.

* * * * * *

44. **PRECISE TERMINOLOGY:** Everyday breakdowns in communication occur. Misunderstandings arise. Clients draw wrong conclusions and people's feelings are hurt. In many cases, the cause is simply a poor choice of words. You say one thing; the client hears something entirely different.
The term girls is belittling, unprofessional, and demoralizing, not to mention chauvinistic. Some clients resent being "turned over to the girls," especially for matters related to patient care. They question if a "girl" is capable. Terms that lead to better communication and have more positive connotations include staff, professional staff, veterinary technician, assistant, office manager, receptionist.

* * * * * *

45. **CLIENT EDUCATION SOLVES PROBLEMS:** Every aspect of veterinary practice can be improved through client education. Client acceptance of the practitioner's recommendations, collection of fees, client compliance with instructions, client respect for office hours or the appointment system, the practitioner's reputation; or number of referrals are common problems.

* * * * * *

46. **QUESTIONS OFFER OPPORTUNITY:** Practitioners who are truly concerned about their clients' total needs neither dodge nor resent questions. Instead, they welcome the opportunity to educate and reassure apprehensive clients.

17

47. **BROCHURE EDUCATES CLIENTS:** To educate his clients, Dr. C.G. Hoover, Seabrook, Texas, has developed a brochure about his **Clear Creek Animal Hospital.** Along with statements regarding clinic policies and philosophy is the following: "Regarding euthanasia: As veterinarians, we are dedicated to preserve the health and well-being of animals. Please do not ask us to terminate the life of an animal with a curable condition".

* * * * * *

48. **TECHNIQUES OF COMMUNICATION:** Never guarantee results of therapy. Even if it were possible to guarantee results, there would still be some people who would be dissatisfied with the situation. Always discuss the prognosis of the disease involved and be certain to mention possible complications of therapy.

Set fees commensurate with the difficulty of the problem involved and the amount of time required. Spell this out beforehand and itemize all bills to show which portion of the fee is for professional services, laboratory studies, radiographs, ECG, and other tests or services.

Do not hesitate to suggest a consultation if the patient or family seems to question your diagnosis or therapy. If you are correct, the consultation will make you look better. If you are wrong, you stand to learn something.

Give the patient's family special consideration. If members of the family are in allied health professions, they are more likely to register complaints.

Be certain that your answering service clearly knows who is substituting for you when you are gone.

Be certain to return calls to clients promptly, especially if the client is dissatisfied with your services or with the results of therapy. It is far better that clients talk to the veterinarian involved than if they talk to neighbors, malpractice lawyers, or a mediations committee. Deal openly and directly with the clients specific complaint.

Think twice before sending a bill to a collection agency, especially if the client has a reason to be dissatisfied with your services. If you encounter clients you cannot learn to like, help them find another veterinarian.

Improve communications, display common courtesy, and practice listening.

* * * * * *

49. **COMMON COMPLAINTS:** The following items concerning grievances were given George Thomas, D.V.M., while serving as

Chairman of Ethics, Professional Conduct, and Grievance Committee, Southern California VMA, 1962:

A. Lack of communication between veterinarian and client invites complaints.
B. Lack of consideration invites complaint. Kindness and patience are, or should be, virtues.
C. Indecision encourage complaints.
D. Excessively high fees invite complaints.
E. Excessively low fees invite complaints.
F. Failure — invites complaints.
G. Release of soiled or dirty pets invites complaints.

Conclusion: A veterinarian must work with the vigor of youth, must act with the wisdom of many years of experience, must always be right, must never fail, must charge reasonable fees, must convey heartfelt interest in the client and his pet, must strive to avoid pitfalls of incomplete communication between the client and himself. When we fail, the Chairman of the Ethics, Professional Conduct and Grievances Committee will be hearing about us. Rots of ruck.

* * * * * *

50. **TAX DEDUCTIBLE:** Clients should be advised that veterinary expenses incurred for dogs kept for the protection of business property are deductible business expenses.

* * * * * *

51. **COLLECTION PROCEDURE:** When a client leaves the office, the receptionist should ask if they wish to pay by cash or by check. If the person indicates he wants to charge the bill, give him a statement of services rendered in a special self-addressed envelope which contains an up-dated statement of his account. Tell him that you prefer not to send a monthly statement. Also, ask him to use the self-addressed envelope to return his remittance. This is an excellent collection device if these two steps are used.

* * * * * *

52. **JUSTICE OF PEACE COURTS:** In Indiana, Justice of Peace courts are highly effective agencies for collecting bad checks and bad debts. A letter to the party involved telling them you are turning the matter over to the J.P. is a highly effective action-producing procedure.

* * * * * *

53. **BURIAL RELEASE:** To assure payment for your services when a hospitalized patient dies or must be euthanatized, request that the

owner come to the hospital to sign the "necessary release" for euthanasia or burial.

* * * * * *

54. **D.O.A. PROCEDURE:** When a client brings in an animal that is dead on arrival, or if a patient succumbs during the examination or preliminary work, always drape the body until it has been removed, or until the client has left the premises.

* * * * * *

55. **RESPECT SHOCKS:** When you have to tell a client shocking news that will severely disturb him . . . dismiss him and talk to him later. While they are reacting to the "blows" it is a waste of time to discuss the matter. The difference between a man with a huge practice and a man with a little practice, is that the first man knows how to handle people so they remain happy, feeling secure and friendly.

* * * * * *

56. **WATCH NIGHT CALLS:** If you must make an emergency trip to your clinic late at night for a client with whom you are not familiar, notify the police either to phone you at the office or have a police cruiser stop by. It's not a bad idea to ask them check at your home while you're away.

* * * * * *

57. **TIPS FOR CLIENTS TRAVELING BY AUTO:** To avoid diarrhea, carry a supply of the water the pet normally drinks. If this is not possible, bottled distilled water should be used. If the animal is prone to car sickness, it should be offered chipped ice. This provides necessary fluid without loading the animal's stomach with liquid. Don't change the pet's diet unless absolutely necessary and feed him in the evening after stopping for the night.

* * * * * *

58. **PRESCRIPTION RENEWAL:** Tourists often request a refill of the pet's medication. Before dispensing anything in these situations, ask the owner to fill out a standard registration form, stating the medication, its use, and the name of the doctor who usually cares for the pet. If the medical situation seems urgent, insist on examining the pet before complying with the request to renew a prescription or dispense other medication. It is sometimes prudent to contact the veterinarian who usually cares for the pet.

* * * * * *

59. **RESPECT ANAPHYLAXIS:** Because of sensitivity of individual

animals to some drugs and biologics, it is good insurance to ask clients to remain with their pets in the reception room or in their cars for a reasonable interval after treatment. When clients are informed that the delay is to make certain their animals have no anaphylactic or allergic reaction, they do not mind the wait. In fact, they appreciate the additional concern shown for their pets.

* * * * * *

60. **DEFINE EXAMINATION:** Legally, an owner's request to check over a dog means only a physical examination. It does not mean laboratory work. The client does not have to pay for laboratory work under this type of arrangement. Be sure the owner understands this when he asks you to examine his animal.

* * * * * *

61. **CAREER GUIDANCE:** A new booklet of special interest to young persons interested in veterinary medicine as a career has been published by the AVMA. Entitled "Today's Veterinarian", the booklet offers excellent general information about the profession. Copies are available in quantity from the AVMA, 930 N. Meacham Road, Schaumburg, Illinois 61072.

* * * * * *

62. **RECEPTION ROOM NEWS:** A bulletin board with appropriate material and placed in your reception area can offer three important benefits to your practice. It can help keep your professional image up-to-date; it can educate your client on a variety of topics; and it can provide recognition for your staff, your clients, and yourself.

* * * * * *

63. **RUBBER STAMP EFFICIENCY:** Save time in giving client instructions which you issue often (*e.g.*, instructions for administration of anthelmintics you dispense) by having the instructions made on a rubber stamp.

* * * * * *

64. **SEND HOME SYRINGE:** To solve the problem of accurate home administration of oral medication to pets, provide the pet-owner with a graduated syringe. The dosage is easy to calculate and administer. Example: A cat weighing 8.8 lb (4 kg) and requiring a medication (100 mg/5 cc) at a dosage level of 50 mg/kg/day in four doses would be given 2.5 cc q.i.d. Our clients have found this drenching technique to be easier and more accurate than using an eyedropper.

65. **INEXPENSIVE BALLING GUN:** To facilitate administration of tablets or capsules to cats, cut the tip off of a 3-cc disposable plastic syringe with a pair of nail clippers. This makes a "balling gun" that can be sent home with the patient to help resolve the problem of giving medication at home.

******

66. **PEANUT BUTTER HELPS:** When clients indicate they cannot give a tablet to a dog, recommend they crush the tablet and mix it with some homogenized (creamy type) peanut butter. The peanut butter sticks to the dog's mouth and teeth and dogs do not resist this method of administration. One word of caution: do not use too much peanut butter.

******

67. **WRAP THE CAT:** To help clients avoid getting scratched while administering oral medication to a cat at home, suggest that the cat be wrapped in a heavy bath towel fastened with a safety pin.

******

68. **TIP FOR CLIENTS WITH A NEW PUPPY:** When the puppy wets on the carpeting, absorb the moisture with a clean, dry cloth or tissue. Cover the damp spot with about ½ inch of salt and leave the salt on until it dries. Pick up the salt with a carpetsweeper.

******

69. **DEODORIZE INDOOR-OUTDOOR CARPETING:** Use 1 cup of Clorox® solution in 5 gallons of water.

******

70. **FLEA CONTROL:** When a dog admitted for hospitalization or boarding is found to have fleas, advise the owner that spraying or dusting the home and the dog's quarters with an insecticide will alleviate the flea problem in the house and greatly aid in controlling the flea infestation when the dog returns.

******

71. **BAGGY TECHNIQUE:** For the client who appears to be squeamish about bringing in a stool specimen, suggest enclosing the hand in a plastic sandwich bag, grasping a bit of the feces, and then inverting the bag and knotting it or closing it with a plastic tie.

******

72. **THUNDER DESENSITIZATION:** To condition a dog that becomes upset during thunderstorms, have the owner get a tape recorder and

equip it with a loop (continuous tape) and record the noise of a severe thunderstorm. The tape should be played back to the dog daily for about an hour, beginning at low volume and gradually increasing the volume on successive days. If necessary, the owner should pet the dog and speak reassuringly to it while the tape is played.

******

73. **PUPPY MANAGEMENT:** Best time to take a puppy from a litter is 7 weeks (plus or minus one week). The puppy has about 3 weeks to socialize with its own kind and at this age it is best for it to socialize with man. If it is taken from the litter too early it becomes antisocial toward dogs. If it is taken from the litter too late it becomes antisocial toward man.

******

74. **EMERGENCY EMETIC:** Hydrogen peroxide is a good, safe, and readily available emetic for a client to give a pet in an emergency situation. Recommend giving one teaspoon orally every 5 to 10 minutes until the animal vomits.

******

75. **CLIENT INFORMATION:** Consider distributing a brief newsletter from your hospital or clinic. It can be mimeographed or duplicated on an office copy machine and mailed to regular clients. Copies should also be made available in your reception room. The purpose of the letter would be to offer seasonal information (*e.g.*, data on heartworm) and to inform clients of absences of the staff to attend continuing education programs; change of hours during holidays; and staff vacation schedules, etc.

Chapter/4

EMPLOYEE RELATIONS

Dedicated and productive employees are the backbone of any good business. This is especially true in the life of a small animal practitioner. Obtaining and keeping good employees is a common problem. We seek employees with intelligence, character and experience but we frequently give little inspiration in return. Good employee-employer relationships are based on mutual appreciation and understanding. Supervise them efficiently but not boldly. Allow them to participate, train them well, outline their duties, and communicate freely. The team work approach works well in veterinary practice. Everyone works together to operate an efficient, well organized hospital for the care of animals. Your staff can and should make your life's work easier. The following practitioner ideas will emphasize the role of a good personal relationship with your employees.

EMPLOYEE RELATIONS

76. **EMPLOYEE FULFILLMENT:** No one denies that money is a powerful motivator, but it is not the only motivator. People respond to recognition and appreciation, to a feeling of belonging and participation, and to interesting, meaningful work that provides a sense of self-fulfillment.

******

77. **TRAINING BY VISITATION:** Much of our success depends on how well our employees understand how to do their assigned jobs. Many employees have never seen anyone else do the work they're doing. Therefore, it is impossible for them to know if they are doing an excellent or a lousy job. Take your employees to visit other veterinary hospitals. Your people will quickly decide if the quality of their work is superior or inferior to that being conducted in other facilities. Important—establish a regular visitation schedule.

******

78. **ADVICE ON HANDLING EMPLOYEES:**
    A. Hourly employees.
       1. These people are not paid to make decisions. Set-up their work in such a way that they are not required to make decisions.
       2. Prepare a work list of what they are to do each day in the order of importance to you. Do not say "Wash the windows if they need it". This requires a decision. Simply require the windows be washed every day.
       3. Supervision is the most important problem you have. Become a prowler to assure that work will be done like you want.
       4. Don't expect them to do more than they are capable of . . . *i.e.* kennel man answering the phone!!
    B. Salaried employees.
       1. Prepare work lists so they can initial each item as they completed.
       2. Supervise . . . supervise . . . supervise!!

******

79. **LOOK SHARP:** When the women employed at the Jefferson State Bank in San Antonio, Texas, were supplied with tailored suits and dresses, the quality of their work and their attitude improved. Each girl was given two jackets and three skirts for winter wear and a different colored dress each weekday during the summer. All girls wear

the same color dress on a given day of the week. An arrangement similar to the Jefferson State Bank is used in an Ohio veterinary hospital. The hospital employees present an outstanding professional image. Why? Because the owner instructs all employees to purchase and charge the necessary uniforms, hose, and shoes to the hospital. Each employee *must* keep his clothes cleaned and pressed and his shoes polished. Everyone is expected to look sharp (haircuts for men; coiffures for women). All of the clothes are of high quality, and the people are proud to be a part of this organization. (Have you looked at your employees' shoes lately?).

* * * * * *

80. **PERSONNEL IDENTIFICATION:** Provide all employees with plastic embossed name tags. This method of identifying personnel seems to improve the doctor-client relationship, as well as employee morale.

* * * * * *

81. **INVITE SUGGESTIONS:** Encourage your staff to offer ideas and suggestions for improving your practice. Whenever possible, make a point of adopting ideas that have merit. The recognition will provide a tremendous psychological lift to your employees.

* * * * * *

82. **JOB ENRICHMENT:** Industrial psychologists say the key to happy employees lies in improving the content of their jobs. This concept of improving a job so that it yields more intrinsic rewards is known as *job-enrichment.*

* * * * * *

83. **BUILD THE TEAM:** Giving "VIP" recognition to the members of your staff is good management psychology. It lets them know they are respected as important members of the veterinary medical team. It boosts their morale and upgrades your hospital.

* * * * * *

84. **THE THREE MAGIC "A's" FOR EMPLOYMENT:** Acceptance, Approval, Appreciation.

* * * * * *

85. **SOCIAL INFLUENCES IMPORTANT:** Hawthorne in experiments found that social influences were more important in the productivity of employees than any other factor. These findings have since been corroborated by other investigators. The influences are:

1. Sense of participation and belonging: Before any changes in the working situation were made, the women were consulted, their opinions solicited.
2. Sense of pride in their work: The women knew they were taking part in an interesting experiment.
3. Knowledge of results: The women were given regular reports of their progress.
4. Improved social relationships: The women worked under conditions free from hard-and-fast supervision. A high level of cooperation, teamwork, and group cohesiveness was developed by the employees.

* * * * * *

86. **CRITICIZE EARLY:** Many veterinarians think the best time to criticize is at the end of the week. They think Saturday is a good time for a heart-to-heart talk about matters that need improvement. Industrial psychologists say this may actually be the worst time of the week. Everyone is anxious to get away. The discussion is hurried, and the employee goes home in the poorest frame of mind possible. Once home, he or she may blow the criticism out of proportion. The weekend is ruined, and by Monday morning resentment runs deep. For best results, time the discussion of a problem so that you have another chance to talk to the employee before the day or week is over.

* * * * * *

87. **THINK BEFORE CRITICIZING:** Nothing is as unfair and upsetting as unwarranted criticism. Even if you apologize later to an employee for assuming that a mistake had been made, the harm has been done. Your actions have shown how little confidence you have in the employee.

* * * * * *

88. **RESPECT DEMANDS PRIVACY:** Never criticize or correct an employee in front of co-workers or clients. The only place to deliver criticism is in your private office, with the door closed. Although this is common sense, it is not common practice.

* * * * * *

89. **BE SPECIFIC:** Nothing can lower morale in a practice as much as an expression of general dissatisfaction without a clear statement of what is expected. Most employees are anxious to "do it right" if they know what "right" is.

* * * * * *

27

90. **FATIGUE IS OUR MOST DANGEROUS AND UNDERESTIMATED ENEMY:** Many receptionists (and veterinarians) suffer fatigue from working too many hours. It's easy to spot these people. They're disagreeable, impatient, critical, and discourteous. Smiling becomes an effort for them. These people often work 50 to 60 hours a week. Why not consider using two people to do their job so that you can have happy, cheerful office personel.

******

91. **WRITTEN PROGRAM HELPFUL:** When hiring a new person, ask him to give you a written program. Allow the person an overnight opportunity to prepare this report. This will provide a challenge. This procedure will weed out those people who are not really interested in the job. A person who is interested in the job will write up what they sincerely think can be done to help the operation.

******

92. **SUCCESS FORMULA FOR HIRING THE RIGHT PEOPLE:**
    A. Character
    B. Intelligence
    C. Experience
Too often, we reverse the order.

******

93. **EMPLOYING RECENT GRADUATES:** Those veterinarians who are employing or anticipate employing recent college graduates should know that the typical college graduate today considers recognition as an individual as important as the size of his paycheck. He is interested in:
    1. The opportunity for growth.
    2. The opportunity for challenge.
    3. A chance to make a contribution to society.
    4. A chance to write his own job description.
It is important to assign him tasks that fit their capabilities and potential. Offer a career that gives a prospect of adventure. Many veterinarians fail to appreciate the fact that recent graduates are expecting to earn between $15,000 and $20,000 on their first jobs. This is a trend of the times. The fact that you worked for $400 a month 20 years ago, doesn't change the situation at all. This means that the employer must be open-minded and realistic regarding all employees, professional and nonprofessional. Otherwise, you'll have a "parade" of employees through your business and you will supply "on the job" training for people who will leave you to work for someone else.

94. **MOONLIGHT HELP:** Use a part time bookkeeper in the evening to handle the bookkeeping paperwork. There are bookkeepers who will work from 6 to 9 p.m. for as little as $3.00 per hour and they are readily available. This relieves the receptionist from bookkeeping and works better for all concerned. An ad in the paper will quickly obtain the services of a bookkeeper.

******

95. **EMPLOYEE ABSENTEEISM:** To reduce employee absenteeism on Mondays, pay on Monday rather than Friday.

Chapter/5

RADIOLOGY

Radiology is a vital tool in the discovery and diagnosis of disease. A basic knowledge of the safe use and interpretation of radiographs is necessary in every practice. It is hard to imagine that a competent practice can exist without radiographic equipment.

Radiology may be broken into the physical and mental components. The physical aspect is the actual preparation of the radiograph. It is important to follow consistent steps in taking and developing radiographs. The mental component is the intrepretation. It is important to have some form of systematic approach to the reading of radiographs. Radiographs that are difficult to interpret should be saved for further consultation. The following ideas and tips cover the entire radiological program in your practice.

RADIOLOGY TIPS

96. **PROCESSING FACILITIES:** Film processing is an important part of quality radiography. Many correctly positioned radiographic examinations are spoiled by improper processing. Proper processing can only be accomplished in an environment that is conducive to careful film and cassette handling. Knowledge of processing technique alone will not insure against poor results if adequate facilities and equipment are not provided.

* * * * * *

97. **DARKROOM ESSENTIALS:** Darkroom facilities must be efficiently designed. You need a "dry bench" area for loading and unloading cassettes, an area for proper film storage, and an area for wet tanks.

* * * * * *

98. **PROTECT FILM:** Purchasing x-ray film in small amounts decreases the possibility of exposure to damaging elements (even when the storage method consists of closing the top of the box in which the film was purchased). Additional protection may be provided by storing opened film boxes in a darkened cabinet. This cabinet should be located a distance from the x-ray machine to avoid exposure to scattered radiation.

Unexposed film should be stored in a room with a temperature between 50 and 70°F. Opened film boxes should be kept at a relative humidity of 30 to 50 percent. Film should never be stored in a drug room or next to sources of formalin, hydrogen sulfide, hydrogen peroxide, or ammonia vapors. Films should be placed on end. Stacking tends to produce pressure artifacts after exposure and development. The oldest film should always be used first.

* * * * * *

99. **CONVENIENT TRANSFER BOX:** For increased efficiency of cassette handling, add a cassette transfer box between the darkroom and the x-ray room. Install this container in the wall for accessiblity from either side. An interlock mechanism prevents inadvertent opening of the box on the light side (x-ray room) while the dark room is in use. This box provides a convenient and readily accessible storage area for loaded cassettes.

* * * * * *

100. **VENTILATION VITAL:** Adequate darkroom ventilation provides an environment free from volatile chemicals. Proper air circulation also helps control temperature and humidity. A light-tight exhaust fan installed in the ceiling, when accompanied by a light-tight air intake

louvre, permits sufficient air circulation. Heater exhausts from film dryers and automatic processors should be vented to the exterior of the darkroom.

******

101. **SPILLS CAUSE DAMAGE:** Periodic cleaning of tank surfaces should be a routine procedure in darkroom maintenance. Wipe up spilled solutions immediately. They evaporate, leaving a chemical dust that may contaminate and damage film and screens.

******

102. **USE VACUUM CLEANER:** X-ray cassettes should be vacuumed and cleaned periodically to eliminate the accumulation of lint.

******

103. **REDUCE EXPOSURE TIME:** When using high speed film (ex: Kodak royal blue) the exposure time can be reduced by approximately 50%. High speed screens reduce exposure time by 25%.

******

104. **FIX FILMS FOR STORAGE:** Radiographs which you have been in a hurry to see and have read when wet may lose their contrast and become discolored. Always return them to the processing tank for sufficient fixing and final washing time.

******

105. **COOL DEVELOPERS:** To prevent fogging of x-ray films, cool the developer solution to 68°F with frozen gel packs (Stay-Cold® or Blu-Ice®). The packs float, are easy to remove, refreeze and reuse. Frozen gel packs can be obtained from shipments of some biologics or can be purchased in the camping supply department of most retail stores.

******

106. **PREPARE LABELS:** Precut several x-ray marking-tape labels to avoid the necessity of measuring and cutting one every time you prepare to take a radiograph.

******

107. **KEEP APRON UP:** To assure optimum protection against accidental exposure to x-radiation, the leaded apron should always be worn well up on the shoulders. Leaded aprons do not provide protection back of the shoulder seam. Thus, when an apron slips forward, direct or scatter rays can penetrate the fabric and strike the wearer.

******

108. **MEASURE WITH STRING:** To facilitate measuring and positioning when taking radiographs, attach a string (equal in length to the proper focal distance) to the tube head of the x-ray machine.

******

109. **MARK VIEW BOX:** To make small radiographs easier to read, use cardboard or paper to mask the illuminated area of the viewing box surrounding the margins of the film, thus reducing the glare.

******

110. **SKETCH LINES:** When reading challenging radiographs, especially those of the abdomen, lay a sheet of Saran Wrap® (or similar material) over the film on the viewer. With a fine or medium-point marking pen, sketch the lines of demarcation around areas of varying intensity. The film is thus preserved and the lesions can be more readily evaluated. The procedure is also an aid in communicating findings to clients and planning corrective surgery.

******

111. **POSITIONING TIP:** Achieving a good radiograph of the anterior border of the heart (using a low power machine) may be assisted by pulling the four legs back along the rib cage of an anesthetized dog.

******

112. **REFERENCE SUTURES:** When conducting a neurological examination for a possible disc lesion, place a stainless steel suture over the suspected problem site before taking radiographs. Measure the distance from the suture to the lesion on the radiograph and leave the suture in place during surgery. This reference-suture pinpoints the area for incision and eliminates the guesswork associated with using the anticlinal vertebra as a reference point.

******

113. **SODIUM IODIDE TRACER:** Chronic fistula of the skin may be traced on a radiograph by injecting sodium iodide solution. Those in the flank area can often be traced to spay sutures Vetafil® (S. Jackson). Inject the tract with gentian violet or other dye before surgical removal.

******

114. **SKY BLUE TRACER** can be injected directly into the esophagus to outline the thoracic duct. It can be injected into the cyst to make sure all the lining is removed. Use a very small needle.

******

115. **FEWER G.I. FILMS REQUIRED:** When taking radiographs of the gastrointestinal tract, administration of Oral Hypaque Sodium® (Winthrop) will decrease the transit time to the cecum, when compared with barium sulfate suspensions. A more rapid identification of gastrointestinal lesions, foreign bodies, or displacement of viscera is possible. When this technique is used, fewer radiographs are needed and less handling of the animal is required.

Chapter/6

LABORATORY

Virtually every disease process can be diagnosed by using analysis and interpretation of body fluids, tissue cells, enzymes or waste products. These tests are forecasters of disease and can aid in the prognosis of disease. Whether you use an outside laboratory or your own facilities, the laboratory is one of the most important diagnostic tools available to practitioners.

Time and cost are of concern. Many tests can be run in your own laboratory facility. Screening tests are now available which offer more dimension in diagnosis and save time. A hospital laboratory facility should contain the necessary equipment to run fecals, smears and enzyme tests, WBC's and blood smears, heartworm tests, urinalysis and sediment examination, kidney function tests, culture facilities both bacterial and fungal, blood analyzer tests (Glucose, SGPT, Total Protein, etc.), and microscopic examination of hair, skin, tissue cells, ophthalmic and genital secretions. Commercial laboratories can supplement testing not available to the practitioner. It is important that the veterinarian stay abreast of new tests available and understand the significance. Your assistant or technician must also be aware of these new tests. They must be able to give you results in all the laboratory procedures. Mistakes here can obscure and change the therapy and diagnosis. The following tips offered will make your laboratory procedures more accurate and practical.

LABORATORY TIPS

116. **USE SOLVENT CONCENTRATE:** To wash dirty glassware and stained syringes use a regular super solvent concentrate (containing methanol) of the type available from service stations. Add 2 oz. of the concentrate to each quart of water and soak the glassware. This process is good for removing greasy smears from slides used for fecal examination.

******

117. **GREASE RELIEF:** To clean your microscopic slides and remove the grease film, use a small amount of laundry detergent and the household product known as Grease Relief® (Texize Chemical Co.).

******

118. **BIZ OR AXION:** "Stuck" glass syringes can be made operational by soaking them in a solution of either Biz® or Axion® presoak detergent and then boiling them in the solution.

******

119. **PLASTIC COVERSLIP HELPFUL:** To facilitate the transfer of a fecal specimen to a slide, use a plastic coverslip on the fecal flotation vial.

******

120. **EASIER VIEWING OF COCCIDIA IN FECAL SMEARS:** Obtain a fecal specimen from the suspected host and smear it on a microscope slide. Allow the slide to air-dry for approximately 10 minutes (no coverslip). Add 2 drops of Difil-Test® (Evsco) to the slide. Coccidia will be apparent under the microscope because they do not stain.

******

121. **ZINC SULFATE:** In the case of chronic diarrhea in dogs, particularly those in a kennel, be suspicious of strongyloides infection. Use a 33% zinc sulfate flotation test to demonstrate the larvae. (excellent for coccidia oocysts, too).

******

122. **PERFORMING BLOOD TESTS FOR HEARTWORM DISEASE:** Collect the blood in a 3-cc syringe. Leave the needle attached and insert the needle into the opening in the tip of a 12-cc syringe. No overflow problem is encountered. This procedure distributes blood well in the diluent in addition to eliminating the use of tubing.

******

123. **TOO MUCH FORCE ALTERS RESULTS:** When using the filter technique for heartworm tests don't force the diluted blood through the filter. Too great a force will push the microfilaria through the holes

in the filter and a positive sample may be called negative.

******

124. **HEARTWORM TESTING OF SMALL BREEDS:** To prevent blood from clotting in the syringe while drawing blood samples for heartworm testing of small or toy breeds of dogs, add 1 drop of stabilized heparin solution to the syringe before performing the venipuncture. The heparin solution is inexpensive and can be obtained in 15-ml dropper bottles.

******

125. **MICROFILARIAE DIFFICULT TO DETECT:** Dogs tested for heartworm may not exhibit microfilariae, but a surprisingly large number will still be harboring adult filariae. For this reason, clients should be advised to start prophylactic doses of diethylcarbamazine with caution and to observe their dogs carefully for any signs of untoward reaction.

******

126. **CORTICOSTEROIDS ALTER LEUCOCYTES:** Any corticosteroid may produce changes in the leucocyte picture of animals. In the horse, the WBC may double and lymphocytes decrease 30% with no change in monocytes. In the cat, WBC may double or triple. In the dog, neutrophils increase three to four times, and lymphocytes decrease 50%, while eosinophils disappear.

******

127. **CHECK BUN AND SGPT:** Prior to giving a dog the arsenic treatment for heartworm, check BUN and SGPT. Never give arsenic if BUN is elevated. If elevated and treated, you can expect reaction. Post-treatment BUN and SGPT are excellent tests to measure toxicity, particularly if you have a "before" reading.

******

128. **WATCH PCV:** Excess excitement of animal can cause physiological neutrophilia and increase the PVC by 10-15%. Excess anticoagulant interferes with stain reaction and can decrease the PVC by 30-35%.

******

129. **CAPILLARY FILLING TIME:** A quick and easy test of capillary filling time can be made by pressing the patient's gums with a finger and observing how rapidly color returns to the blanched area. (Normal: rapid, pink. Abnormal: 1 to 5 seconds, membranes still gray.)

******

37

130. **VOMITUS ORIGIN:** To determine if vomitus is from an esophageal or a gastric obstruction, check the pH. If it is very acid, it is from the stomach.

* * * * * *

131. **DEMONSTRATE EAR MITES:** Mineral oil introduced into an ear with a pipette can be aspirated to demonstrate ear mites under the microscope for the client.

* * * * * *

132. **OXYDEX® AIDS SKIN SCRAPINGS:** A small amount of Oxydex® (Dermatologics for VM Inc.) shampoo gently rubbed onto the area before taking skin scrapings helps in finding sarcoptes mites because keratinaceous debris is broken down.

* * * * * *

133. **PLACE SLIDE ON MICROSCOPE LAMP:** When making skin scrapings for ectoparasites, the parasites can be made more active, and thus more readily visible, if the slide is warmed on the microscope lamp for a minute or two prior to microscopic examination.

* * * * * *

134. **COMPLETE URINALYSIS INVALUABLE:** The kidney is an inarticulate organ - the bladder is its voice box - time spent in a complete urinalysis is the most valuable time spent in the laboratory.

* * * * * *

135. **GRAM-NEGATIVE BACTERIA:** Most bacteria cultured from urine of blockage patients is gram-negative.

* * * * * *

136. **DIAGNOSTIC AID:** When dealing with urinary tract infections, Bacturcult® (Wampole) is an excellent diagnostic aid for urine culture, bacterial count, and presumptive bacterial-class identification. The small plastic tubes provided with this system can even be incubated at room tempeature. Results are evident in one or two days.

* * * * * *

137. **CYST STERILE:** If a culture is made of an early interdigital cyst before it ruptures or before it has been debrided, the lesion's contents are usually sterile. This would not be the case with primary pyodermas, mycotic lesions, or lesions caused by mites.

* * * * * *

138. **OLIVE OIL INCREASES GROWTH:** Pityrosporum canis can be

isolated from cases by culturing on Fungassay Dermatophyte Test™ medium (Pitman-Moore). Growth may be increased by the addition of a few drops of sterile olive oil prior to inoculation. Incubation at 25 °C for 2 weeks is recommended.

******

139. **LABORATORIES REPORT RESULTS:** Outside laboratories report results of tests. They do not diagnose. They cannot and should not suggest treatment for any problem brought to light by a particular test.

******

140. **RESPONSIBLE FOR DIAGNOSIS AND THERAPY:** The practicing veterinarian is responsible for the examination, diagnosis, and treatment of his patients' disorders and may be held liable for unwarranted or erroneous diagnosis and therapy. The veterinarian cannot evade the responsibility by attempting to delegate that responsibility to a laboratory.

Chapter/7

PHARMACY

A practitioner may write prescriptions instead of dispensing the indicated medications but they will still find it necessary to stock preparations for use in treating hospitalized animals. Specialty items not available in the drug stores of the community should be included in this stock. A veterinary pharmacy should have a sufficient quantity of fresh drugs, easily located. A convenient system of inventory control is needed so that replacement stock can be ordered in time. An indication of the cost of these items for proper billing is important.

Major divisions of the drug room or pharmacy should provide space for insecticides (powders, dips, sprays), parenteral fluids, controlled drugs, and bulk items. Shelf space is best organized according to therapeutic purposes (antibiotics, cardiac, urinary, etc.). Drawers or shelves are needed for dispensing paraphernalia (safety vials, bottles, labels, etc.), and sufficient counter space is needed so medications can be packaged and labeled.

Shelves should be systematically numbered or lettered with every item assigned a specific area. The proper organization of the pharmacy helps when a relief veterinarian is there as well as when you ask your aide to bring a specific item.

Records are important and a log of all controlled drugs dispensed is mandatory. An inventory (other than that necessary for controlled drugs) will show turnover and what items could best be bought in greater quantity. All products should be marked or coded either on the bottles or on an index card. This can be kept simple. Some list cost and purchase date (*e.g.* 10-1275-79 = bought October '79, cost $12.75), others add dispensing fee (*e.g.* 20/2 = 20 for $2.00) and some code purchase price (*e.g.* 1234567890 MYTS = $12.75).
MY HOSPITAL

Proper labeling of all medications dispensed is important and must list owners name, animal, instructions, medicine, amount, proper warning of any risk, doctor's name and date.

John Doe, DVM
1234 Main Street
Anytown, NY 12345

F. Harris dog Cleo
One Capsule every
8 hours.
15 Ampicillin 250mg
9/30/79

For Veterinary Use Only

PHARMACY TIPS

141. **DRUG INVENTORY CRITICAL:** The current problem of drug abuse makes it more important than ever that veterinarians maintain careful control over their drug inventories and drugs they dispense. Recent news stories indicate that sodium pentobarbital euthanasia preparations dispensed for veterinary use are now a threat on the drug scene. One teen-ager in Kansas City, Missouri, has been hospitalized with apparent brain damage, and another has died after ingestion of a pentobarbital preparation intended for enthanasia of horses.

* * * * * *

142. **FDA REGULATIONS AFFECT VETERINARIANS:** The FDA has many regulations that directly affect veterinary practitioners. You should review all the regulations with special regard to who can count tablets or capsules, the type of containers that must be used for dispensing various types of medications, the need for a signed consent form when child-proof containers are not dispensed, and what drugs must be kept under lock and key.

* * * * * *

143. **ADVISE CLIENTS ON PRESCRIPTION REFILLS:** Permitting unlimited prescription refills is poor medical practice. Owners of animals with chronic conditions (cardiac, skin, etc.) should be advised as to how long a prescription can be refilled before the patient's condition must be re-evaluated.

* * * * * *

144. **KEEP RECORDS:** Keep a record of the number of tablets dispensed for a patient. It can be vitally important if the client's child accidentally ingests the medication.

* * * * * *

145. **UNIVERSAL PADLOCKS:** Keeping all drug cabinets locked when you are not on the premises often necessitates carrying a large assortment of keys. To overcome this inconvenience, have simple clasps installed on the cabinets and order padlocks that can all be opened with the same key.

* * * * * *

146. **USE OLDER DRUGS FIRST:** To make certain older drugs with an expiration date are used first, mark all items put into the pharmacy with a number indicating the sequence in which they are to be used.

* * * * * *

147. **COLORED FILE CARDS:** As a time saver and extra safety measure, use a file card of a different color for animals that show a reaction to drugs.

148. **LABEL MEDICATION:** When dispensing medication, always write the animal's name or the name of the owner and the animal on the container. If anyone suffered ill effects from accidentally taking medication from an improperly labeled container you dispensed, you could be held liable.

* * * * * *

149. **ASK BEFORE DISPENSING:** Before dispensing a topical medication that could stain furniture or carpeting, check with the client to determine where the pet sleeps.

* * * * * *

150. **EXTENDED USE OF VIALS:** Avoid repeated puncturing of the stopper on a multiple-dose vial of a parenteral preparation by inserting a needle and cap with a removable needle plug that is left in the stopper.

* * * * * *

151. **INVERT BOTTLES BEFORE USE:** When using injectable penicillin and similar preparations that require considerable agitation before use, be sure to invert the bottles differently each time after use. This simple precaution insures that the particles remain in suspension and do not settle out.

* * * * * *

152. **REFUND FOR BACK ORDERS:** When ordering large quantities of drugs from wholesale suppliers, always ask for a refund check covering the cost of any back-ordered items. This frees your money so that you can purchase the needed drugs elsewhere. It is also a good idea to photostat all orders before they are mailed.

* * * * * *

153. **WATCH DRUG COSTS:** Cost of drugs and therapeutics (not including expendable equipment) should be around 15% of the gross income. If this percentage goes up it is time to reduce your drug costs or to adjust fees. This % may vary with other types of practices.

* * * * * *

154. **GLASS BOTTLES AVAILABLE:** A source of glass bottles for dispensing is the mortician. Most morticians have a large supply of suitable bottles (originally containers for embalming fluid) which they are pleased to have carried away.

* * * * * *

155. **LABEL PHARMACEUTICALS:** When labeling glass jars used to store

43

pharmaceuticals, use labeling tape on the front of the jar to identify the drug and write the price per capsule or tablet on the inside of the jar lid. This saves time when you must determine the price of individual items in the pharmacy.

******

156. **SIMPLE TABLET DIVIDER:** A quick and easy way to divide tablets into halves or quarters is to use a White nail trimmer. The nail trimmer makes dosing for small animals more accurate and the tablet almost never crumbles.

Chapter/8

ANESTHESIA

Today's trend in anesthesia is divided between the newer, injectable, anesthetic combinations and inhalation anesthesia. Preanesthetic medication with tranquilizers and/or narcotics is still commonplace and may be useful for the stressful patient. This may also assist endotracheal intubation or may make "masking down" with inhalation anesthetics possible. Atropine is still given as a preanesthetic and to overcome bradycardia. The safety and effectiveness of nitrous oxide as an adjutant to inhalation anesthesia has been much debated. Nitrous oxide is still considered useful in the complete inhalation anesthetic system.

The neuro-lepto-analgesics and combinations of these drugs are playing a more active role in total anesthesia. One of the trends is getting away from barbiturate usage and switching more to the neuro-lepto-analgesics. Drugs like ketamine and Rompun® (Haver Lockhart) are becoming more a part of the current style. However, the mainstay for prolonged anesthesia today are the inhalation anesthetics like methoxyflurane and halothane. This trend will probably continue.

A thorough working knowledge and comprehension of any of the anesthetics you use in your practice is important. The following practice tips are typical of some newer anesthetic trends.

ANESTHESIA TIPS

157. **COMPLACENCY BREEDS TROUBLE:** When we become complacent about anesthesia, we are in for real trouble. Anesthesia is, at best, only a means of temporarily controlled poison.

******

158. **WARNING!!!** Animals without any body fat can develop prolonged respiratory arrest after intravenous Surital® (Parke-Davis) solution or any barbiturate solution.

******

159. **ANESTHESIA CAN BE REDUCED:** If you have a narcotics license, keep a supply of 6-mg apomorphine hydrochloride hypodermic tablets on hand. They come in handy if a dog has been fed or if there is doubt about its having been fasted prior to abdominal surgery. One tablet dissolved in 1 cc to 2 cc of sterile water and injected subcutaneously will cause vomiting within 10 to 15 minutes in a 20-lb dog. After this treatment, the dosage of anesthetic can be reduced.

******

160. **CONVENIENT STORAGE:** Tape an old case from a plastic syringe to your gas anesthetic machine to store a syringe for inflating the cuff of your endotracheal tube.

******

161. **PREVENT ACCIDENTS:** When a syringe is taped to a dog's leg, slip rubber tubing of small diameter over the ends of an Allis forceps and clamp one end of the forceps on the syringe barrel and the other end on the plunger. This device keeps the syringe from filling with blood or being accidentally pushed in.

******

162. **USE INTRAVENOUS TUBING:** A quick and clean method of adding the solvent to a 5-mg vial of Surital® (Parke-Davis) is the use of intravenous tubing attached to a 1,000-cc bottle of sterile saline solution. Two 1-inch, 20-gauge needles are inserted through the rubber stopper; one to relieve pressure and the other to receive the tubing.

******

163. **GREYHOUND AND WHIPPET SEDATION:** Combine equal parts of Vetame® (Squibb) 20 mg/ml and Num Orphan® (Endo Labs) 1.5 mg/cc ml. Give intravenously or subcutaneously at rate of 1 ml/10 lbs., up to 5 cc.

******

164. **SAMPLE FROM JUGULAR VIEN:** When taking a blood specimen from a cat, try withdrawing it from the jugular vein. In order to calm the animal before starting the procedure, give 0.25 cc of ketamine intramuscularly.

******

165. **MINIMUM RESTRAINT:** Give cats 0.5 cc of Demerol® (Winthrop) subcutaneously 20 minutes before administration of an intravenous anesthetic. Using a 26-gauge, 3/8 inch needle for the intravenous injection, a minimum of restraint is required.

******

166. **CHEMICAL RESTRAINT:** For chemical restraint of cats, mix 2 cc promazine in 10 cc ketamine. Give 0.1 cc/lb body weight plus 0.1 cc.

******

167. **INCREASE RELAXATION:** To achieve a greater degree of relaxation in patients given ketamine, add 1 cc of 10 mg/ml Acepromazine® (Ayerst) to 10 cc of 100 mg/ml ketamine. Give the recommended dose of ketamine. Be sure to label the vial containing the new mixture.

******

168. **PLUGGED-UP CATS:** It may be too dangerous to use ketamine in plugged-up cats. Since you do not know the status of the kidneys unless tested, it is far wiser to use tranquilizers, local anesthetics, nitrous oxide, oxygen, and inhalant anesthesia for short periods.

******

169. **ALTER BEHAVIOR:** It has been reported that Psymod™ (Pitman-Moore) is a valuable tranquilizer in terms of truly modifying feline behavior. A dosage rate of 1 mg/ 5 kg of body weight is recommended. Psymod™ can be administered either orally or parenterally.

******

170. **MOOD MODIFIER:** Psymod™ is an excellent mood modifyer and sedative. Often will quiet down barking dogs, mean cats, etc., without much tranquilization. Good single anesthetic in old animals with kidney disease . . .helpful in unplugging cats with FUS (Feline Urinary Syndrome.)

******

171. **ADMINISTER INNOVAR-VET™** intravenously with equal parts of 1/120 gr. of atropine in 1 ml of Innovar™ (Pitman Moore) for 30 to 60 lbs. of body weight. Excellent for C sections . . . can tube with above

dose and use Metofane™ (Pitman-Moore) or nitrous oxide. After trimming a dog's ears and removing from anesthetic machine, give 1 ml/60 lb. interveneously to prevent thrashing . . . not necessary to give atropine twice. For hip dysplasia, give large dose if painful . . . narcotic wears off in about 20 minute. Can give Nalline® (Merck) as last resort for mobility.

******

172. **EASE PASSAGE OF ENDOTRACHEAL TUBES:** Inject ketamine in cats and Innovar-Vet™ (Pitman-Moore) in dogs. Both drugs are given with atropine. The dose of ketamine is 5 mg/lb intravenously. The dose of Innovar-Vet™ is 0.1 cc/5 lb intravenously. We have found these drugs to be safer than the standard, short-acting barbituarates and post-operative recovery to be faster. According to the manufacturers there is no reaction between these drugs and methoxyflurane.

******

173. **COATHANGER WIRE:** To facilitate passage of an endotracheal tube in a cat, use a length of coathanger wire as a stylus. The wire can be easily autoclaved and the end bent back to eliminate the sharp point.

******

174. **MOUTH GAG AVAILABLE:** A mouth gag for intubating cats is readily available in the form of the hard container used for packaging the Monoject® needle/syringe combination unit (Sherwood Medical Industries). When the needle and syringe have been removed, the case provides exactly the same tool described by Dr. Fowler in the May 1972 issue of vm/sac (p 470). Saving these cases offers a ready supply of mouth gags with no extra cost or effort involved — and you can afford the luxury of single-patient use.

******

175. **MOUTH GAG FOR INTUBATING CATS:** Drill a hole of appropriate size in the barrel of a 3 cc disposable syringe. A power drill works best but a bone pin also works well if it has been preheated with an autoclave. (A cold pin will crack the plastic.) A hole made with a 1/8-inch pin readily allows passage of a No. 10 French catheter, and this size works well for adult cats.

******

176. **LOCAL ANESTHETIC SPRAY:** Spray Cetacaine® (Haver-Lockhart) to make passage of an endotracheal catheter much easier.

******

177. **INTUBATING DOGS OR CATS:** With animal in dorsal recumbency, have an assistant grasp the larynx through the skin of the neck and push the larynx forward. Grasp the fold of tissue beneath the epiglottis with 9 inch Doyen or Scudder intestinal forceps in the mouth and pull forward. This makes intubating very easy.

******

178. **INDUCING ANESTHESIA IN DOGS:** Use a combination of Rompun® (Haver-Lockhart) and Ketaset® (Bristol). Give a subcutaneous injection of 1 mg Rompun® /1 lb bodyweight. The dog will vomit. After five minutes, give 75 mg Ketaset® /10 lb bodyweight, intramuscularly. The dog will be ready for surgery in five to seven minutes. Allow the same dosage rate of Ketaset® for dogs weighing up to 30 lb, but never give more than a 300-mg total dose to larger dogs. Adopting this technique, gas anesthesia equipment will be virtually unused.

******

179. **SIMPLIFY ADMINISTRATION:** An excellent anesthetic combination for cats is Rompun® (Haver-Lockhart) given subcutaneously, followed in 15 minutes by intramuscular injection of Ketaset® (Bristol). In a vaccine diluent bottle, prepare a solution by adding 1 cc of Rompun® to 5 cc of saline, sterile water or diluent. The resulting concentration is approximately 17 mg/cc. For subcutaneous dosage at 1 mg/lb, administer 0.5 cc of this solution. When the cat has been preanesthetized in this way, about 0.25 cc of Ketaset® (25 mg) is sufficient for ovariohysterectomy, castrations, etc. Preanesthetize dogs with Rompun® given subcutaneously at a dosage of 1 mg/lb. This is followed by intravenous administration of pentobarbital at about half the normal dose level. These combinations of anesthetics have been used without untoward reactions. Rompun® given subcutaneously is tolerated by fractious animals. In cats, the normally irritating Ketaset® is accepted intramuscularly without resistance. The muscular rigidity caused when Ketaset® is given alone is not seen after preanesthetization of the animal with Rompun®. Surgery cases can be admitted in the morning and released late in the afternoon of the same day.

******

180. **SAFE AND EFFECTIVE:** A new anesthetic combination of ketamine Rompun® works best when given together in the same syringe intravenously with atropine. The dose is .1 - .2 cc of each per 10 lbs given with ½ cc - 2 cc atropine intervenously. This mixture is safe and useful for short surgical procedures and compatible with inhalation

49

anesthetics for longer surgical procedures. It works well in the dog or cat. Double the dosage and give the mixture subcutaneously for longer surgical procedures.

******

181. **DISPOSABLE FACE MASKS:** If you use the drip method of administering inhalation anesthetics, paper Dixie® cups of different sizes with holes punched in the bottom make good disposable face masks.

******

182. **AVOID EXCITEMENT:** To avoid the excitement phase in a canine patient anesthetized with pentothal sodium, give 1/5 to 1/4 dose of Sparine® (Wyeth) during the recovery stage.

******

183. **REVERSE DEPRESSION:** To reverse severe depression from shock or overdosage of anesthetic in a cat, immerse the animal up to the head in water at about the temperature used for a hot bath. Many animals respond immediately to this treatment. To prevent chilling, the patient is toweled dry and wrapped in a newspaper cocoon.

******

184. **IMPROVE VENTILATION:** For respiratory depression in dogs and cats, tie a piece of 3 inch gauze bandage tightly around the chest cage. This will cause a prompt improvement in ventilation.

******

185. **PAIN INCREASES RESPIRATION:** In a dog that is breathing shallow during a prolonged post-operation period, a deep breath caused by pain (*i.e.*, sharp squeeze behind stifle or pinching toe) will greatly aid in respiration response.

******

186. **IMPROVE RESPIRATION:** Calicium gluconate, 0.5 cc/lb given slowly intravenously may be a useful analeptic in sleepers by improving respiration, heart action, and liver function.

******

Chapter/9

SURGERY

The primary consideration in surgery is the life and well being of the patient. Age and the health of the animal and time and cost of surgery often play significant roles in determining if surgery will take place. As practitioners, we must be certain we are benefiting both the client and the patient with surgery. To endanger a patient's life when surgery is of little benefit is inappropriate.

To insure success and profit with surgery, a surgeon must be systematic and consistent in his attitude toward surgery. Preliminary exams on all surgical patients is essential. CBC's, serum protein and blood urea nitrogen tests are necessary. Intubation and administering anesthetics that you are familiar with is important. Monitoring vital signs during surgery is necessary to avoid emergencies. Administering intravenous fluids and preventing chilling during surgery have proved to be life-savers. Following surgery, administration of oxygen is beneficial, especially after long surgical procedures.

Finally, the surgeon should set aside a certain time in his practice solely for surgery. This prevents interruptions and provides adequate time should complications arise. The best surprise is no surprise. The best success is to have an animal leave the hospital in better health than when it was admitted. The following tips will benefit both the surgeon and the patient.

SURGERY TIPS

187. **NO SYMPTOMS - NO SURGERY:** It is difficult to make the asymptomatic patient better with surgery.

******

188. **ELECTIVE SURGERY:** If elective surgery is scheduled fairly well in advance, it is wise to call the day before and remind them. At this time, you can request the animal be bathed before being brought into the hospital for surgery.

******

189. **GENERAL PURPOSE ELECTROLYTE:** Lactated Ringer's is an excellent general purpose electrolyte solution for intravenous use. It is also excellent for flushing out the abdominal cavity (add antibiotics when necessary).

******

190. **FREE FLUIDS:** Hospitals often destroy large amounts of outdated fluids. These are often satisfactory for use in animals and can be obtained for hauling them away.

******

191. **WARM FLUIDS:** To avoid shock when administering fluids that are too cold, keep all fluids used for therapy in an incubator immediately prior to use.

******

192. **EMERGENCY SITUATIONS:** To save precious seconds in emergency situations, keep emergency parenteral solutions (*e.g.* epinephrine, nalorphine, anesthetic antagonists, etc.) in sterile syringes provided with a needle guard and clearly labeled.

******

193. **STERILE WATER:** Keep on your surgical tray a 2-oz (or larger) jar of sterile water. (Run it through your autoclave cycle when instruments are being sterilized.) Dip suture material in the water to wash off the preservative. A gauze sponge dipped into the water can also be used to wipe talcum off the outside of new surgical gloves.

******

194. **AN ALTERNATIVE TO ETHYLENE OXIDE FOR STERILIZING ENDOTRACHEAL TUBES:** Place the tube in a closed container together with an open jar containing 30% formaldehyde. Leave the tube in the container for eight hours.

******

195. **AUTOCLAVE PAPER TOWELS:** Sterilize a small package of paper towels by autoclaving. A paper towel often comes in handy during surgery and these autoclaved towels can be used without breaking sterile technique.

******

196. **KEEP TRACK OF GAUZE PADS:** When preparing surgical packs, always count out gauze pads in multiples of 5 or 10. Using a set number of these pads during surgery helps account for any that might have gone into the abdomen after tissues have been packed (as in cesarean section, cystotomy, etc.)

******

197. **EASILY OPENED:** When preparing surgical packs (instruments, gloves, etc.) fold about 0.5 inch of the autoclave tape over itself so that the packs may be opened easily.

******

198. **ECONOMICAL:** To save time and autoclave tape, use masking tape for most of the sealing and then place a small strip of autoclave tape on the pack to serve as a marker.

******

199. **SURGICAL PACK PREPARATION:** To make the preparation of surgical packs easier, keep a card file or notebook of the surgical procedures you perform. List for each procedure the instruments, special supplies, number of sponges, etc. you require. This is a great help to the technician who prepares your surgical packs.

******

200. **MARK SURGICAL PACKS:** When sterilizing packs of sponges, gloves, etc., mark the date on the autoclave indicator tape to assure use of the packs in correct sequence and to provide a check on appropriate quantities to be pre-sterilized.

******

201. **GLOVING CREAM:** Use Bisorb Gloving Creme® on the hands before putting on surgical gloves. It works better than talcum powder. It comes in individual packets and is available from Arbrook Co., Koley's Medical Supply.

******

202. **REUSE SURGICAL GOWNS:** Disposable surgical gowns need not be discarded after they have been used in surgery. They make excellent

protective overgarments for use in the kennel area when painting or other especially messy chores must be performed.

* * * * * *

203. **STERILIZE AND REUSE:** Many human hospitals discard disposable items which are still suitable for reuse in the animal hospital. Check with your local hospital for endotracheal catheters, surgical glove packs, suture materials, etc., that you can resterilize and use.

* * * * * *

204. **INTRAVENOUS STORAGE:** To store a rubber simplex intravenous outfit after it has been cleaned and sterilized, roll it to fit into a 6 7/8" × 7 3/4" Waxtex sandwich bag. To seal, just roll down the open end of the bag and staple shut. This type of pack can be stored safely in a practice case or drawer until needed.

* * * * * *

205. **DACHSHUND INFUSION:** The Butterfly® Infusion Set-21 (Abbott) is valuable for use with dogs that have short, crooked legs (*e.g.*, Dachshunds). The set provides a fine plastic tubing with a syringe adapter on one end and a thin-walled, 21-gauge needle on the other. The needle can easily be taped to the animal's leg.

* * * * * *

206. **ECONOMICAL AUTOCLAVE:** An economical autoclave can be purchased from Sears in the form of a heavy case aluminum pressure canner.

* * * * * *

207. **RECOMMENDED BY MANUFACTURER:** An excellent aid in the care of blades for both large and small animal clippers is a solution made up of 1 part light motor oil to 2 parts of kerosene. While the clipper is running, submerge the blades in the solution. After heavy use of clippers, soak the blades in the solution overnight. Oster recommends this kind of care.

* * * * * *

208. **STICKY SIDE OUT:** To prevent cotton wadding from slipping when preparing a padded splint, wind adhesive tape around the splint with the sticky side out.

* * * * * *

209. **IMPROVISE:** A Schroeder-Thomas Splint is sometimes less irritating to a dog if the inner portion of the ring is completely smooth and left

54

unpadded. An effective material for making Thomas Splints for cats and small dogs is galvinized clothesline wire or rubber-coated copper electrical wire.

* * * * * *

210. **REDUCE CONSTRICTION AND COMPRESSION** of the toes when applying a Thomas Splint to the leg of a small animal by slipping a plastic spool from a roll of adhesive tape over the foot before taping the splint into position.

* * * * * *

211. **TO REMOVE LIGHTWEIGHT PLASTER CASTS:** Affix a used No. 22, Bard-Parker® blade to a No. 4, Bard-Parker® handle. With the aid of a needle-holder or pliers, break the blade off at the tip of the handle. This leaves a short, strong, square-end cutting tool that is unlikely to slip or skid on the first few cuts. With repeated passes, a deep cut can be scored into the cast.

* * * * * *

212. **REMOVAL OF CASTS:** To facilitate removal of a plaster cast, imbed a Gigli Saw in the cast, leaving the ends exposed.

* * * * * *

213. **TUBING PROTECTS SAW:** To prevent the rusting of a Gigli Saw wire imbedded in a plaster cast, insert the wire into old plastic intravenous tubing when the cast is applied.

* * * * * *

214. **STOCKINETTE MAINTAINS APPEARANCE:** Cover the splint on a fractured limb with a stockinette. It produces a more professional appearance while preventing involvement of debris with the tape and keeps the splint looking better for future use.

* * * * * *

215. **PREVENT ANIMALS FROM CHEWING ON CASTS:** Use concentrated quaternary ammonium solution daily on the cast or the bandage. This solution is very bitter, and animals will avoid it.

* * * * * *

216. **DELAY BANDAGING:** Dr. Ruggles suggests that you delay the bandaging of the surgical wound for 3-4 hours, if at all possible, to allow the wound to air dry.

* * * * * *

217. **ECONOMICAL CAST-SPREADER:** For an efficient cast-spreader at

one-tenth the cost of a conventional medical cast-spreader, use Cock-ring Pliers (Powercraft Tools, #84-7454). This device easily separates either plaster or fiberglass.

* * * * * *

218. **DISPOSABLE GLOVES OFFER VERSATILITY:** Vinyl disposable gloves protect the patient and the doctor. Use them when tattooing, applying iodine, methylene blue or any other preparation where staining may be a problem.

* * * * * *

219. **SURGERY POSITIONER:** To make a positioner for patients undergoing surgery in dorsal recumbency, tape together two 500-cc bottles, leaving about 4 inches and a saddle of tape between them. This positioner will comfortably accommodate most dogs weighing from 10—20 pounds. For toy breeds, 250-cc bottles may be used.

* * * * * *

220. **COMFORTABLE DISTANCE:** When performing canine surgery, strap the animal on the table at a distance which is most comfortable for you rather than always centering the body on the table.

* * * * * *

221. **EFFECTIVE LIGHTING:** Heavy duty fluorescent tubes as used in gas stations are useful in examining rooms and surgery.

* * * * * *

222. **ECONOMICAL INSTRUMENT STANDS:** Feeding trays that roll over the bed in human hospitals make good instrument stands . . sturdy . . buy used.

* * * * * *

223. **EFFICIENT USE OF RAZORS:** For longer and more effective use of preoperative surgical razors, use separate blades for dogs and cats.

* * * * * *

224. **VERSATILE STERILE JELLY:** Before clipping the hair around a wound that must be cleaned, fill the wound with water-soluble sterile jelly. This simple procedure keeps hair out of the wound and makes it much easier to clean. The jelly also lubricates the clippers.

* * * * * *

225. **HEAT SOURCE:** A light bulb placed under surgery table is an effective and inexpensive source of heat.

226. **KEEP DRY AND CLEAN:** A wire-mesh platform (drying rack) placed under a dog while ultrasonic dental procedures are being performed will help keep the animal dry and clean about the face.

* * * * * *

227. **EFFECTIVE ANTISEPTIC:** Routinely spray isopropyl alcohol after standard scrubbing procedures. It is nice to know that alcohol is still the *best* antiseptic on the market and you probably will never see a skin reaction to it.

* * * * * *

228. **SIMPLE APPLICATION OF A STAINING SKIN ANTISEPTIC:** Spray the antiseptic from an 8-oz bottle equipped with a plunger-type sprayer.

* * * * * *

229. **ETHER IMPROVES STICK:** An economical and efficient way to make adhesive tape stickier for use on splints, ear trims, etc., is to spray it with commercial-grade ether used to help start motors (available in aerosol cans).

* * * * * *

230. **VERSATILE:** Often a small disposable drape is needed for suturing a lesion or for a simple surgical procedure. The paper in which surgical gloves are folded in the package is good for this purpose. If care is taken in opening the package, contamination of the paper can be avoided. When you have finished using the gloves, wash them while they are still on your hands, dry them, apply Johnson's Baby Powder®, and remove them. They make inexpensive nonsterile exam gloves. If you are right-handed, turn the left glove inside out.

* * * * * *

231. **AUTOCLAVED STOCKINETTES:** Many veterinarians are using autoclaved stockinettes to cover the entire leg of dogs and cats prior to fracture repair. This is the simplest and easiest way to cover the entire leg with sterile material. It greatly decreases the chances of contamination during bone pinning and other surgical procedures. The sterile stockinet can be rolled over the leg that has been clipped and scrubbed.

* * * * * *

232. **AUTOCLAVE PLASTIC ITEMS:** If you encounter shortages of plastic items and disposables such as syringes and needles, try washing and autoclaving them. Most of these items will stand up very well under this type of "recycling".

233. **AUTOCLAVE INTERNAL SUTURES:** Any Vetafil® (S. Jackson) used as an internal suture should be autoclaved rather than chemically sterilized. Never store internal sutures in a liquid disinfectant.

******

234. **EASY TO HANDLE:** For surgeons that use stainless steel sutures . . . try using 4-0 multifilament (not monofilament) for standard abdominal closure. It is much easier to handle and you can even tie a surgeon's knot with it.

******

235. **SURGICAL SCRUB:** Add approximately 2 cc Nolvasan-S® to Nolvasan® shampoo (Ft. Dodge) to make your own Nolvasan® surgical scrub.

******

236. **BLOOD STAIN REMOVAL:** To remove blood stains from a dog or cat after surgery or a blood venipuncture, wash the area with Septisol Surgical Soap® (Vestal) or hydrogen peroxide. This practice is especially pleasing to the owner of a white-haired animal.

******

237. **GIVE ANTIOBIOTICS BEFORE SURGERY** . . not after . . so there will be a level in all devitalized tissues.

******

238. **ADVANTAGES OUTWEIGH DISADVANTAGES:** Pre-operative and intra-operative intravenous administration of a balanced salt solution such as Lactated Ringer's Solution will help maintain adequate blood pressure and reduce the incidence of postsurgical renal failure. The advantages of intravenous therapy during surgery far outweigh any disadvantages in cost or time.

******

239. **A NEW METHOD OF ABDOMINAL AND THORACIC PARACENTESIS:** An indwelling intravenous catheter is used for the tap. To locate fluid, air is injected through the catheter while the abdomen or thorax is auscultated and the operator listens for a diagnostic "bubbling" sound. The main advantages of this method over the older method using a hypodermic needle are that a negative tap is truly diagnostic of the absence of fluid, fluid is easily located and sampled, and the risk of injuring intra-abdominal or thoracic organs is minimal.

******

240. **WHEN INSERTING A PENROSE DRAIN,** use a stab incision and an-

chor the drain away from the line of incision. This procedure minimizes the licking of the suture line. The drain can also be removed before the incision has completely healed.

******

241. **ELIMINATE HEIMLICH VALVE:** An excellent chest drain for cats with empyema and other thoracic surgeries is a K-61®, sterile suction catheter, size 10 French (Pharmaseal). Be sure to cut at least two more holes near the end for better drainage. You can repeatedly drain the chest and eliminate the need for a Heimlich Valve.

******

242. **LIFE SAVER:** In cases of diaphragmatic hernia in cats, a considerable degree of atelectasis may be present as a result of pressure from the abdominal viscera. Many cats can be saved by tracheal intubation followed immediately by inflation of the lungs with gentle bag pressure.

******

243. **WHEN DOING A PHARYNGOTOMY** in those animals that need oral supplementation, suture the stomach tube or catheter to the skin. After a couple days the animal can be sent home with the tube in place. Pass a smaller tube or catheter thru to give your food and medication. A drop or two of Biosol-M® (Upjohn) on the tongue will keep vomiting under control if a problem.

******

244. **CROPPING A PUPPY'S TAIL:** Use a "V" ear notcher of the type used for cattle. This will leave the flaps necessary for suturing.

******

246. **LEFTOVERS:** Left-over absorbable sutures with small swaged needles can be resterilized. They are excellent for closing the flaps when you dock the tails of puppies.

******

246. **EPHINEPHRINE MINIMIZES BLEEDING:** When docking tails or dewclawing young pups, a drop of epinephrine to the incised area will decrease bleeding.

******

247. **BACTERIAL CONTAMINATION:** Operators of ultrasonic teeth cleaning machines should be aware of the danger of bacterial contamination from the atomized mist produced during cleaning. Masks should be worn and the machine kept out of surgery areas.

248. **IMPROVED ELEVATOR:** The regular tooth elevator is improved with a V notch (fine three cornered file) in the end of the elevator.

******

249. **EXTRACTION OF CANINE CARNASSIAL TOOTH:** Wrap adhesive tape around part of a new hack-saw blade to form a handle. Saw transversally across the upper carnassial tooth down to the gum line until tooth splits into two sections. This 3-rooted tooth can be extracted easily.

******

250. **USE TOWEL CLAMP FOR ALIGNMENT:** While seating the pin when reducing a fractured mandibular symphysis in a cat, the jaw can be best held in alignment with a towel clamp.

******

251. **TRAUMATIC SEPARATION OF THE MANDIBLE IN THE FELINE:** Half hitch stainless steel wire over the lower canine teeth, and secure it posterior to the symphysis by tying the wire on a button over the skin. You should have normal approximation of upper and lower jaws when sutures are pulled tight. Remove in about 3 weeks. This procedure leaves no scar and there is no drainage. Some animals immediately start to eat. This is an excellent procedure if there is no fracture but separation of skin from the mandible is evident.

******

252. **REDUCE UTERUS BEFORE SURGERY:** Surgery in cases of canine pyometra-metritis is safe and simple, if, before surgery, 0.2 to 0.5 mg of ergonovine maleate is given intramuscularly every other day for three treatments. Schedule surgery one week after the first office visit and treat the dog as an outpatient during that time. Clinical improvement is marked after the second injection. The size of the uterus is almost normal at the time of surgery. Administration of antibiotics and supportive treatment in conjunction with the ergonovine is optional. Surgery is mandatory since the condition always recurs.

******

253. **INCISION SITE:** To find the site of incision for the flank approach to ovariohysterectomy in a cat, put the cat on its right side. Place your right thumb on the point of the greater trochanter, and your right middle finger on the pelvic ilium. Put your right forefinger on the flank of the abdomen so that the finger is one point of an equilateral triangle formed in combination with the middle finger and thumb. The tip of the forefinger marks the center of the incision line.

254. **EFFECTIVE TECHNIQUE:** To minimize frustrating mishaps while performing an ovariohysterectomy, try the following procedure: After completing a routine laparotomy and exposing one of the uterine horns, break down the ligamentous attachment to the ovary. Dissect a hole in the broad ligament to allow passage of a suture around the ovarian vessels. Use forceps to clamp the uterus caudal to the ovary. Do not apply more clamps. Palpate for the ovary and gently elevate it from the incision. (This is a job for an assistant if one is available.) Elevation of the ovary should expose an area of the ovarian vessels that can be ligated. Use a fairly heavy synthetic suture material such as Vetafil® (S. Jackson) for litigation. Double-ligate the vessels under as little tension as possible. Using blunt-tipped scissors, resect the ovary, cutting carefully between it and the ligatures. Repeat the process on the other side of the uterus and, after tying off both uterine vessels, remove the uterus by cutting through the body. Do not ligate the uterine vessels between clamps or above or below a clamp. Be sure to tie the sutures with as little tension as possible.

The objective is to ligate the vessels while they are in a natural relaxed state. This eliminates the danger of cutting through vessels while tying sutures next to forceps or of sutures slipping off when the forceps are released. An added advantage is that the ovary need not be elevated from the incision as much as is normally required. Resection of the ovary while holding it in the fingers gives the added assurance that all of the ovary is being removed.

****

255. **CANINE C-SECTION:** Assure continuous oxygenation of the puppy by delivering it from the uterine incision with the umbilical cord and placentation intact. The fetal membranes are cleared from the head and torso and the airways cleared by gentle suction with a sterile rubber spiration bulb.

As soon as spontaneous ventilation is established, pulsations in the umbilical vessels will diminish. The cord may then be ligated or clamped.

If it is clamped, use light weight metal or plastic clamps made for this procedure.

The weight, shape, and general clumsiness of a hemostatic clamp across the cord predisposes undue traction. The latter can result in intra-abdominal tearing of the umbilical artery-vein and may weaken the ring. Post-natal umbilical herniation may occur.

******

61

256. **MINIMIZE RESPIRATORY DEPRESSION:** For cesarean section in the bitch, give a preanesthetic of morphine sulfate and atropine, followed in 20 minutes with apomorphine subcutaneously. No additional anesthetic is required, no respiratory depression occurs, and the pups will nurse within 30 minutes.

* * * * * *

257. **RELAX LIGAMENTS:** To relax the ovarian ligaments when performing ovario-hysterectomies, inject 2 cc of 2% lidocaine intraperitoneally.

* * * * * *

258. **BETTER RANULA RESULTS:** When doing a ranula operation, incise and suture the inner layer to the mucous membranes and leave as an open area.

* * * * * *

259. **CYTOTOMY FOR SMALL CYSTIC CALCULI:** Use a sterile 50-cc syringe filled with isotonic saline solution and attach to a short flexible catheter. Direct solution into the urethra from the bladder to flush through any small calculi that may be lodged in the urethra.

* * * * * *

260. **PACKING A DOG'S OR CAT'S EYES, NOSE OR JAW AFTER SURGERY:** Use a small (6-inch diameter) English ice bag. It's just the right size and costs only $1.75.

* * * * * *

261. **ICED RINGERS** help in back and bone surgery by reducing bleeding, swelling, and oxygen needs of the tissue. This is helpful in the healing of fractures and in preventing post-operative complications.

* * * * * *

262. **BEND BONE PIN:** Providing a slight bend in the intramedullary pin can afford greater stability and less rotation of the bone.

* * * * * *

263. **MINIMIZE SOFT TISSUE TRAUMA:** Grind or file the protruding end of the intramedullary pin smooth before setting it back under the skin.

* * * * * *

264. **TREATMENT OF HERNIATED DISCS:** Excellent results have been obtained with one proteolytic enzyme tablet, Papase® (Warner Chilcott) three times daily and ultrasound. The ultrasonic treatment is given for three minutes daily for five days and then every other day un-

til an additional five treatments have been administered. The dosage is 0.4 watts per cm². Treatment should begin as soon as possible. Muscle massage and exercise are also beneficial.

******

265. **TECHNIQUE FOR CORRECTING FRACTURE OF THE VEN-TRAL ASPECT OF THE 7TH LUMBAR VERTEBRA:** Place an appropriately sized pin through the wing of the ilium, then through the dorsal spine of L-7.

******

266. **REDUCING A COXOFEMORAL LUXATION:** Make a skin incision over the greater trochanter. Put two, deep, tight mattress sutures of medium or heavy non-absorbable suture directly over the trochanter. This procedure produces pressure that may help prevent recurrence of the luxation.

******

267. **REGROOVING THE FEMORAL TROCHLEA ON CHRONIC LUX-ATING PATELLAS:** (especially those troublesome poodle knees). Use a round rat-tail file designed to sharpen chain saws. These files are available in several diameters appropriate for dogs of different sizes. The resulting groove is anatomically correct in contour and has a smooth articular surface.

******

268. **ASYNCHRONOUS BONE GROWTH:** Angular deformity of the foreleg or a suspected premature closure of one or more of the growth areas of the radius and ulna: Always include the elbow joint in the radiological examination. If incongruency is present due to asynchronous growth of the radius and ulna, surgical treatment of the area should be the first objective since the leg is already shorter than the normal one. It is best corrected by osteotomy of the shortened bone and lengthening to restore congruency of the elbow joint. Osteotomy of the radius and ulna to correct angular deformity is the second objective. Total correction in most cases is usually a two-step surgical procedure.

******

269. **EAR CROP HEALING:** To avoid the crinkling or contraction that can occur as the cut edges of cropped ears heal, tape both sides of the ears and bridge them so that the tips of the ears are about 1 inch apart. Advise the client to apply tension to the bridge and gently stretch the ears at least twice a day.

270. **HEMATOMA MEDICATION:** Following arual hematoma surgery, apply Pellitol™ (Pitman-Moore) ointment to the inside of the external ear before bandaging. It retards the growth of bacteria and fungi and reduces itching which may cause self-mutilation of the surgical area. Pellitol™ contains resorcinol, bismuth, zinc oxide, calamine, and juniper tar. Its non-antibiotic formulation reduces the possibility of bacterial resistance.

****

271. **DR. SCHOLL'S® FOOT PADS:** In postoperative care of an ear trim, the application of Dr. Scholl's® foot pads to the inner surface of the ear often gives a better stand to the ears.

******

272. **BETTER EAR STAND:** Tape the plastic needle guards from disposable syringes to the recently cropped ears.

******

273. **IRREGULAR WOUNDS:** When preparing to close an irregular wound or when making a skin flap, temporarily approximate the edges with Michel Clips to see if further trimming is necessary and to determine the best site for the sutures.

******

274. **NO SUTURE REMOVAL:** For the final suture when performing spay surgery, use 00 or 000 Dexon® (American Cyanamid) as a subcuticular stitch. This can help reduce your workload because the patient need not return for suture removal.

******

275. **SUTURES EASILY DETECTED:** Some years ago I removed some superficial skin lesions from a circus animal and was asked to use skin sutures similar in color to the animal's hair so that people viewing the animal would not be upset. Conversely, I often use sutures of different color from that of a patient's skin and hair because clients are remiss in returning animals on time for removal of sutures. After considerable regrowth of hair the sutures should be easy to find.

******

276. **ACCESSIBLE POSITION:** When catheterizing a tom cat, apply an Allis Tissue Forceps to the prepuce after the penis has been exposed. This simple technique keeps the penis in an accessible position.

******

277. **A FAST, ECONOMICAL AND DEPENDABLE METHOD OF DE-CLAWING CATS:** Under anesthesia, clip off all nails with a Resco nail clipper. Apply gauze and, using autoclave tape, extend a pressure bandage up the leg 5 inches distoproximally. Postoperatively, give Combiotic® (Pfizer) and Bicillin® (Wyeth) intramuscularly. Remove the bandages 5 to 12 hours later to enable the cat to lick and clean the surgical area.

After one day of hospitalization, the patient is released and allowed to return to its normal environment. Continual licking of the wound by the cat will promote rapid, granulation-type healing, outweighing any benefit of prolonged bandaging.

* * * * * *

278. **DECLAWING:** Extend the claw by grasping it with an Allis Forceps. Using this technique, the pad cannot be cut accidentally. The use of White Nail Clippers with this procedure is preferable.

* * * * * *

279. **CONTROL BLEEDING:** Finger cots are a useful aid in bandaging a cat's feet after declawing. Medicated powder is applied, the finger cot slipped over the foot and secured with tape. The finger cots help control bleeding and facilitate removal of the bandages.

* * * * * *

280. **WOUND PROTECTION:** Oral chloramphenicol solution, Bemacol® (Beecham), has broad antibacterial properties and a terribly bitter taste. These characteristics make Bemacol® an excellent medication to apply locally to an inflamed incision after surgery. The drug can also be dispensed in small dropper bottles for application by the client.

* * * * * *

281. **CASTRATING A CAT:** Anesthetize the animal with 0.2 cc Rompun® (Haver-Lockhart) and 0.2 cc Ketaset® (Bristol) intramuscularly. Avoid the damp cage and odor of urine caused by the animal's voiding during the recovery period by putting the cat into the cage without a pan or solid bottom. Set the cage in a grooming tub. The cat usually recovers sufficiently to be placed into a regular kennel within three to four hours.

* * * * * *

282. **NECROPSIES ENHANCE CLIENT RELATIONS:** You owe it to yourself and to your clients to necropsy all medical or surgical cases

that die or are ethanatized. Necropsy is an educational process that sharpens technique and enhances client relations where permission to necropsy is granted.

******

Chapter/10

MEDICAL TIPS

Medical tips are medical abstracts applied to veterinary medicine. They may be direct advice concerning therapy or medical conclusions drawn from observation and scientific fact. They differ from treatment tips in that they provide you with only the medical data and may or may not have specific therapeutic value. Only your interpretation and application of these ideas can determine this. The following medical tips come from a variety of medical opinions and facts. They may change your approach to certain clinical problems or they may give you the ideas and interest to pursue these problems further.

MEDICAL TIPS

283. **THE KEY** to preventive medicine is anticipation.

******

284. **PREVENTIVE MEDICINE:** The single most important factor which has increased the average life span of dogs and cats is the control of infectious diseases by vaccination.

******

285. **UNCOVER THE HEAD:** When using a blanket for the protection of the pet and the veterinarian, the animal may struggle if the head is covered. This distress can be relieved by uncovering the head.

******

286. **SLATTED FLOOR:** To reduce urine-scalding or soiling of patients that are incontinent, paraplegic, or carrying a urinary catheter, place patients in cages with a drying rack or a slatted wood floor. A slatted floor is also advantageous when dealing with animals that have diarrhea or with pups that soil themselves with feces while caged.

******

287. **MASK ODOR:** To remove the unpleasant odor in the examining room and on the patient when expressing anal glands, apply a few drops of diluted Roccal-D® (Winthrop) or Nolvasan® (Fort Dodge) to the cotton before expressing the glands.

******

288. **GREASE YOUR THERMOMETER:** Alleviate resentment of small animals to the insertion of a rectal thermometer by storing thermometers in diluted water-soluble lubricant (1 part lubricant to 6-10 parts water). This also makes thermometers easier to clean.

******

289. **TRASH CAN:** A diaper pail serves as a suitable waste receptable in the examination room. It is easy to clean, easily lined with plastic garbage can liners, and has a spring-loaded self closing lid. Deodorant blocks that fit into the lid are also readily available from any diaper service.

******

290. **RUBBER BAND TOURNIQUET:** Venipuncture on small pets that are fractious or have crooked forelegs is readily accomplished by using a rubber band as a tourniquet. It is small, compresses the vein without tissue distortion, does not slip, and once the needle is secure, is simply cut.

******

291. **TO REUSE VETRAP®** (3M Co.), roll it on the protective cover from a

60 c.c. syringe. The syringe cover makes an excellent core. Its larger end easily accommodates the finger for winding and its surface permits less slippage of the roll than does the original cardboard core.

******

292. **VERSATILE COAT HANGER:** If you are in a pinch for an IV stand, a common wire coat hanger with the arms compressed and bent in a "U" will serve as an excellent emergency stand. It can be hung on a cage, wire runs, or from the ceiling.

******

293. **CARDBOARD COLLARS:** Disposable collars for dogs and cats can be made easily from cardboard pizza pie plates. These plates can be obtained in bulk from a pizzeria at nominal cost.

******

294. **WARM PUPS:** Rejection of a pup by the bitch is caused by low skin temperature in the pup. Rejected pups should be warmed (but not too fast) before they are put back with the mother.

******

295. **PUPPIES DEHYDRATE** seven times faster than adult dogs with the same type of illness.

******

296. **KEEP SMALL PUPS** from stepping in their food and water dishes while confined in a cage, by placing the dishes in the back of the cage.

******

297. **GOATS MILK** is an excellent substitute for bitch's milk.

******

298. **OBESE GERIATRIC PATIENTS:** Dr. Jack Knowles suggests the following program:
   A. Examine and weigh the patient.
   B. Give the patient weekly muscular injections of chorionic gonadatrophin.
   C. Give 150 to 1,500 units, depending on the size of the patient.
   D. Use a reducing diet along with the hormone procedure.
Note: The chorionic gonadatrophin is a heterologous protein and may cause anaphylactic reactions.

******

299. **STRESS OF HOSPITALIZATION:** Old animals with debilitating diseases should be given extra vitamins/hormones and digestive enzymes.

300. **OLDER ANIMALS LACK RESERVE:** Production of stress beyond the older patient's ability to withstand adversity results in failure. Reaction and recovery are slower.

General Principles of Hospitalization of Geriatric Patients:

    A. Allow owner to leave familiar blanket or toy.
    B. Provide quiet surroundings.
    C. Provide bedding.
    D. Feed two or more times daily.
    E. Exercise three times daily.
    F. Check on water intake and urine flow.
    G. Groom frequently.
    H. Introduce a familiar voice as frequently as possible.
    I. Observe behavior.

******

301. **RADICAL THERAPY:** Don't forget to use a radical therapy program to change the biochemical pattern of the chronic patient. For example:

    A. Sex steroids (estrogens) have been used to treat anestrus with good results. This procedure simply restarts the cycle.
    B. Obesity . . . . a 48 hour fast followed by high protein low carbohydrate (low calorie diet) will change the biochemical pattern.
    C. Other examples in medicine are firing and blistering for lameness in horses, insulin or electrical shock for mental problems, intravenous formaldehyde for chronic infections.
    D. Massive doses of corticosteroids intravenously in severe endotoxin shock.

******

302. **PICKLE THE STINKERS:** For dogs that have come in contact with odors that you cannot wash off; after bathing, rinse animal with warm vinegar water. This does not apply to dogs with skin disorders.

******

303. **CHEER® DETERGENT** will clean and brighten the coats of dirty white dogs and cats.

******

304. **ANAL SAC SECRETIONS:** The offensive odor of anal sac secretion is due to organic acids and esters. These compounds are more labile and soluble in alcohol than in water. Thus, when an exam room "accident" occurs, isopropyl alcohol should be used in deodorizing and in the initial decontamination of fabrics and surfaces.

305. **SAVE MONEY AND TIME:** Feeding dogs and cats out of paper disposable trays saves money, time, and cuts down on diarrhea.

* * * * * *

306. **LACTOSE INTOLERANCE** causes diarrhea in many dogs and cats after they drink milk or eat milk products. The problem can be eliminated by adding to the milk or milk products the lactase enzyme Lact-Aid® (Sugarlo Co.).

* * * * * *

307. **CHOKE COLLARS:** Some people walk an aggressive dog with a choke collar that may cause a chronic tracheitis. To take pressure off the trachea, put a loose collar or lead around the dog's flank and run the end through the regular dog harness to the strap back of the front legs. When such a harness is pulled as in a dog pulling on a lead, pressure is applied to the back of the front legs and not on the trachea. Also, the loose "bellyband" often decreases the desire of the dog to pull on the lead.

* * * * * *

308. **POTASSIUM LOSS:** Dogs lose three times as much potassium in vomition as does man. Potassium loss may produce behavioral changes and poor appetite in a dog. Sodium loss causes decreased movement and weakness.

* * * * * *

309. **PET CAT:** Veterinarians interested in feline practice should have a pet cat around the hospital for people to see. This cat advertises to all that people in this hospital like cats. The word will spread.

* * * * * *

310. **ANNUAL PHYSICAL:** Many small animal practitioners do not understand that owners of hunting dogs are great prospects for annual physicals for their dogs. These men are as concerned with the health of their dogs as people owning house pets. It is often necessary to prepare a separate statement for these men as they do not want their wives to know what they spend on dogs used in their hobby.

* * * * * *

311. **BAKING SODA:** Topically it can be applied to itchy feet and skin. For itchy feet, mix 3 tbsp. per quart of water and soak feet. For skin, apply it as a paste over hot spots and itchy skin. A combination of baking soda and vinegar is helpful in removing porcupine quills. The solution softens the lime/calcium deposits in the quill. Soak 15-20 minutes. Bak-

ing soda is an effective antacid and is useful in kidney failure when given in the patient's drinking water. Use 1-2 tsp. per quart of water. A mixture of ½ baking soda and ½ salt is an effective method for brushing a dog's teeth.

******

312. **INEXPENSIVE HOT WATER BOTTLE:** The frozen ice packs that are shipped with vaccines can be thawed out and heated to make useful "hot water bottles". Heat in hot or boiling water.

******

313. **STIMULATE THIRST IN A DOG OR CAT:** Drop a little Vetrado® oral electrolyte solution (Armour Pharmaceuticals) on the animal's tongue. One or two drops may be sufficient. This treatment is more effective than salting the food heavily or putting salt on the tongue.

******

314. **90% OF DOGS WITH SKIN PROBLEMS** have alkaline urine with albumin.

******

315. **DERMATOLOGICAL DISORDERS** in which the animals exhibit hair loss, redness and sloughing of the skin around the axilla and groin are due to an iodine deficiency caused by all meat diets.

******

316. **ALCOHOL REMOVES DNP:** Use plain rubbing alcohol to remove DNP stains from hands and dog's skin, etc. (saturate well and rub).

******

317. **EFFECTIVE INSECTICIDE:** Combination of boric acid crystals and sugar sprinkled around the wards will kill roaches and palmetto bugs and is harmless to all other animals.

******

318. **REMOVE CAREFULLY:** Twisting or pulling off ticks leaves their mouth parts embedded in the skin. The best method of dislodging ticks is to hold a lit cigarette near the back end of the pest. The tick often becomes uncomfortable enough to release its grip. If you don't smoke, a small drop of camphor or nail polish often does the trick.

******

319. **REDUCE BACTERIAL GROWTH:** Pellitol™ (Pitman-Moore) ointment is helpful in reducing bacterial growth in anaerobic areas such as under a cast or following ear or wound bandaging. It is also useful in

protecting skin around the areas frozen by cryosurgery.

******

320. **SYNERGISM:** Penicillin is synergistic with kanamycin just as strep-tomycin is and can be routinely given as a broad spectrum antibiotic. The penetration of kanamycin is improved after penicillin since the cell wall of the bacteria is destroyed by it.

******

321. **TOPICAL ANTIBIOTICS** include crystalline penicillin, tetracycline, and a bacitracin-neomycin-polymyxin B sulfate mixture dissolved in normal saline. Neomycin sulfate may also be mixed 1 mg/ml in 100 ml of saline.

******

322. **ONION POWER:** In a recent study of the bacteria-killing powers of 150 different herbs and plants, the National Onion Association tells us that the ordinary onion was the most potent destroyer of germs. It seems a raw onion when chewed for five minutes or so renders the lin-ing of both mouth and throat completely sterile and destroys harmful bacteria present. Chemical make-up of the onion is quite complicated, but in the future onion-derived germ-killers and therapeutic prepara-tions may be widely used.

******

323. **FLUSH AFTER SURGERY:** The plasma protein Canalb™ (Pitman-Moore) may be helpful in flushing out severly traumatized tissue and the necrotic area following extensive surgery by supplying locally an available form of glucose and amino acids to the cells. Mix Canalb™ (5-10 cc) with a bacteriocidal antibiotic and flush through the wound following surgery.

******

324. **ANTIEMETIC:** A new product in the human field, Trimethoben-zamide HCl, Tigan® (Roche), is an excellent antiemetic for dogs weighing 20 lbs or more. A 100 mg suppository quickly stops the vom-iting. Note: The product may be too toxic for toy breeds or other dogs weighing less than 20 lb.

******

325. **INCREASE INTAKE:** Water added to dry food (crumbled) will in-crease intake 20%. Twenty-five percent (25%) meat added to dry food will increase caloric intake 20%.

******

326. **CANINE GOUT SYNDROME:** High uric acid content in joint fluids causes these problems:

    A. Osteochondritis dissecans.

    B. Eosinophilic panosteitis.

    C. Lick ganuloma.

* * * * * *

327. **MALPRESENTATION:** It is normal for approximately 40% of puppies to be presented posteriorly.

* * * * * *

328. **CHANGE OF SURROUNDINGS** may cause cessation of labor for as long as four hours.

* * * * * *

329. **EXCESSIVE MATERNAL INSTINCT** may occur in old dogs and nervous dogs with small litters.

* * * * * *

330. **LACTATING BITCHES** should be supplemented with vitamin C. Signs of Vitamin C deficiency are increased irritability.

* * * * * *

331. **INCREASE EJACULATION:** Oxytocin increases the number of spermatozoa per ejaculate by 45% when given 5 to 10 minutes before ejaculation.

* * * * * *

332. **TO AUSCULTATE A DOG** of one of the high-strung toy breeds that often go into a state of panic when put on the examination table, put the stethoscope on the animal's chest while it is held in the client's arms or lap.

* * * * * *

333. **CHECK THE TEETH:** In the older dog showing signs of a cardiac problem, skin condition, etc., check to see if the condition is being aggravated by teeth that need to be cleaned.

* * * * * *

334. **WHEN EXAMINING AN ANIMAL'S EYES OR EARS,** a couple of drops of topical anesthetic, such as tetracaine or Ophthaine® (Squibb), help make the patient more tractable and easier to examine.

* * * * * *

335. **CHECK THE PH OF EAR EXUDATES** with nitrazine test paper. If

the specimen is acid, treat for allergy; if alkaline, treat for bacterial infection.

******

336. **CHECKING FOR SKIN OR EAR MITES:** Use Sebumsol® (Parlam), a cerumenolytic agent, on the slide to dissolve the debris and make the mites easier to find.

******

337. **SLIDE SHOW IMPRESSIVE:** Many itchy ears, especially those with greyish or chocolate-colored debris, are caused by mites. Showing the client these mites under the microscope can be very impressive. When treating the condition, dispense a miticide and a soothing agent, such as Panalog® (Squibb), to be used alternately morning and evening. The soothing agent relieves the irritation caused by mites and, sometimes, by the miticide.

******

338. **INSPECT FOR MITES:** When examining coon dogs, always inspect for ear mites. The mites may keep the dog from barking on the trail.

******

339. **QUICK DIABETES TEST:** A test for suspected diabetes when no urine specimen is available is to round off a Labstix® (Ames) at the glucose position and place it under the eyelid. At a level of 180% or higher blood glucose is present in the tears. If the blood glucose is high, there will be a color change.

******

340. **ADRENAL-ANDROGEN DYSFUNCTION:** Male dogs that attract others or squat to urinate are suspects of adrenal-androgen dysfunction.

******

341. **SIAMESE CATS** rarely get steatitis, chronic dermatitis, or miliary dermatitis.

******

342. **AFFECTS HAIRCOAT:** In excess estrogen (*i.e.*, sertoli, hypoandrogenism), the head and feet are the last to lose hair.

******

343. **DIFFERENTIATE:** A rule of thumb for diagnosing skin problems is that symmetrical lesions indicate an internal problem; asymmetrical lesions indicate a topical problem.

******

344. **SKIN TESTING:** When doing intradermal skin testing for atopic disease in dogs, the use of 0.02 to 0.04 ml of test solution is advised. Injection of 0.1 ml of test suspension can give a false positive reaction.

* * * * * *

345. **CHECK THE SKIN:** In attempting to differentiate between hypothyroidism and Cushing's syndrome in the dog, check the skin. The skin of the dog with hypothyroidism tends to be thick; the skin of the dog with Cushing's syndrome will be thin and show a loss of normal elasticity.

* * * * * *

346. **FALSE POSITIVE:** Previous use of antihistamines or corticosteroids may cause a false positive reaction when skin-testing for allergies. Antihistamines may modify a response for 72 hours after they have been administered. Steroids have a much longer negative effect. A dog administered cortisone for six months should be off the drug for six weeks before skin-testing is done. A two-week interval between steroid therapy and skin-testing is usually sufficient if the steroid was given for only four to six weeks.

* * * * * *

347. **TONSILS REVEAL LYMPHOMA:** In cases of canine malignant lymphoma the tonsils have a large, cauliflower-like appearance.

* * * * * *

348. **SIGNALS TUMOR:** Bloody fluid in the abdomen of a cat often means a tumor is present.

* * * * * *

349. **BRUCELLOSIS IN DOGS:** The type of canine brucellosis first diagnosed in Beagles in Canada, England, and several areas of the United States has spread to all states and has been diagnosed in several breeds. The disease may cause sterility or abortion, or result in the birth of severly debilitated puppies.

* * * * * *

350. **TOXIC TREE:** Be aware of the toxicity of the Golden Chain tree to animals. This popular ornamental tree bears long racemes that, together with the bark, leaves, and pealike seeds, contain the alkaloid cystine. Many cases of intoxication, some fatal, resulting from ingestion of parts of this tree have been reported in Britain. Clinical signs include gastrointestinal disturbance, convulsions, and coma.

* * * * * *

351. **REVEALS LAMENESS:** The wear of the toenails will be an aid in locating an obscure leg lameness in a dog. Use a stethoscope on the hip, stifle, and elbow of a dog to aid in diagnosing joint fractures and pathology.

* * * * * *

352. **FLANK MUTILATION:** Cats and dogs often mutilate their flank area when an arthritic area is present in the lumbar or hip skeleton.

* * * * * *

353. **SIGNS OF LAMENESS:** Lameness in the dog is typified by a shift of weight to the sound limbs. If there is a unilateral lameness in either the forelimbs or hindlimbs, there is a dropping of the body when the sound leg is placed on the ground and an elevation of the body when the lame leg is placed on the ground.
Forelimb lameness is characterized by head bobbing. The head is raised when the lame leg is on the ground and dropped when the sound leg is supporting the body.
Hindlimb lameness is characterized by a dropping of the forequarters as a result of overreaching by both forelimbs and by maintaining the head at a lower position than normal. Some breeds raise their tails when a lame hindlimb is on the ground and drop it when the sound leg is on the ground.
When examining the dog for lameness consider the following characteristics: (1) fluidity and coordination of movement; (2) head and tail movement and position; (3) asymmetry between the contribution of the right and left forelimbs and hindlimbs; (4) dropping of the forequarters or hindquarters and (5) arching of the back.

* * * * * *

354. **SURGERY OPTIONAL:** Cats with hip dislocation or broken femoral head often form false sockets easily . . . surgery is not always necessary.

* * * * * *

355. **MANNITOL FOR DIURESIS:** Mannitol 20% solution, 400 mg/lb is a good diuretic and does not cause the rebound that urea does.

* * * * * *

356. **WATCH PROTEIN AND SODIUM LOSS:** Be careful when removing ascitic fluid from a dog on a low sodium diet. Protein and sodium loss produces shock.

* * * * * *

77

357. **ADEQUATE VITAMINS:** B-vitamins may be destroyed in the sterilization of commercial cat foods. Adding raw meat or liver twice weekly insures adequate vitamin sources. Add fat (corn oil) to dry food diets.

* * * * * *

358. **MAY CAUSE BLINDNESS:** Cats fed only dog food may develop hypovitaminosis A and go blind.

* * * * * *

359. **REDUCE PHYTIC BINDING:** Soak dry dog food for about 20 minutes to reduce phytic binding of minerals.

* * * * * *

360. **ARSENIC KILLS HEARTWORMS:** Arsenic destroys the gut of the adult worm. After administration the worm dies from starvation.

* * * * * *

361. **SAFE ANTIBIOTICS IN KIDNEY FAILURE:** Chloramphenicol, cephalothins, erythromycin, Lincocin® (Upjohn), ampicillin, penicillin and doxycycline. Penicillin and Gentocin® (Schering) are synergistic. This combination is the most effective to date. This is especially useful for deep wounds. Penicillin is effective for anaerobic bacteria while Gentocin® is effective for aerobic bacteria.

* * * * * *

362. **ENEMA LIQUID:** Diluted Lubrivet™ (Pitman-Moore) solution is a perfect enema liquid. It can be used with Fleet™ (Pitman-Moore) enema equipment and it can be made as thick or thin as required.

* * * * * *

363. **DON'T FORGET THE NECROPSY KNIFE:** There is nothing in practice that can be as informative as a well conducted necropsy.

* * * * * *

364. **DELAY ENTHANASIA:** In many instances, it is advisable to delay euthanasia until the following day. Often, the veterinarian will decide to treat rather than destroy. Financial return from therapy is much more rewarding than the usual euthanasia fee.

* * * * * *

365. **NECROPSIES ARE INFORMATIVE:** Necropsies are essential in determining the etiology of an illness. Where diagnostic laboratory necropsy rooms are not available, field necropsy should be performed immediately after death. Gross observations should be noted at the time of necropsy and proper tissue sampling made. Samples should be re-

frigerated for bacteriological culture, frozen for virus isolation, and preserved in 10% formalin for histopathology. Containers such as wide mouth glass jars or plastic whirl-pack bags are essential for preservation.

******

366. **AFTER DECLAWING A CAT:** Apply No. 1 tube gauze over the paws. This product not only makes a very neat bandage but is effective for controlling post-surgical hemorrhage.

******

367. **EFFECTS OF STARVATION:** Acute starvation produces a yellow liver; chronic starvation produces a very dark liver.

******

368. **LAST BREATH:** Every animal or human that dies gasping for breath has pulmonary emphysema.

******

Chapter/11

TREATMENT TIPS

Treatment tips are therapeutic ideas shared by colleagues. For the practitioners who have taken the time to write down these tips and ideas, we are grateful. Especially when these ideas save time, money, or help in the diagnosis and treatment of disease. By sharing these practice pointers, we all benefit.

Everything from administering medication, unplugging obstructed cats, treating eyes, ears, skin problems, intestinal disorders, kidney and internal disease, and exotic medicine are discussed. We take pride in offering this wealth of knowledge to you.

TREATMENT TIPS

369. **BALLING GUN FOR CATS:** Cut the needle end from a disposable tuberculin syringe so that the rubber tip of the plunger protrudes slightly when the plunger is fully depressed. Make two notches on opposite sides of the cut end and round the edges. To use, wedge the tablet into the notches and depress the plunger.

* * * * * *

370. **EASES ADMINISTRATION:** Administration of a pill or capsule to a cat: Restrain the front feet with masking tape or have the client or an aide hold the cat's forefeet. After the forefeet have been restrained, stand to the right of the patient and grasp the nape of the neck anteriorly toward the ears. Slowly rotate the cat backwards, keeping its rear on the table and elevating the forequarters until the oral cavity is vertical. Holding the pill or capsule between the right forefinger and thumb, use the middle or ring finger of the same hand to open the cat's mouth by applying downward pressure on the lower incisors. Drop the medication deep into the middle pharynx and continue to hold the head in the vertical position until the medication has been swallowed. When demonstrated for clients, this technique is impressive — especially to those who have tried unsuccessfully to give oral medication to a cat at home.

* * * * * *

371. **ONE-MAN METHOD:** A one-man method for restraining a cat to give oral medication is to grasp the loose skin between the cat's ears and with the ball of your hand or wrist press down firmly over the cat's shoulders, tilting its head backward. The mouth can then be opened easily with the index finger and the pill pushed gently over the cat's tongue without danger of being bitten. The front claws can present a hazard, though, if the cat is unruly.

* * * * * *

372. **CAN'T OPEN MOUTH?** The administration of oral medication to cats can be made easier by first giving Psymod™ (Pitman-Moore) either intravenously or subcutaneously. Give 1/3-1 cc Psymod™ and wait 5-15 minutes. Avoidance behavior and significant muscle relaxation will occur to allow passage of the medication.

* * * * * *

373. **COAT WITH BUTTER:** When administering capsules or tablets to cats, coat the capsule or tablet with butter or margarine.

* * * * * *

374. **LUBRICATE CAPSULES:** When working cats with mixed anthelmintics such as Vermiplex™ (Pitman-Moore), do not use capsules larger than the 2.5 lb size and lubricate the capsule with a small amount of K-Y® sterile jelly. The cat offers less resistance and the possibility of the capsule getting lodged in the pharynx is minimized.

* * * * * *

375. **FORCEPS EASE ADMINISTRATION:** To keep your hands out of the reach of a cat's claws when administering medication, pull the animal's head back and open its mouth. Then grasp the tablet or capsule with large-animal dressing forceps and insert it in the cat's mouth.

* * * * * *

376. **DISTRACT PATIENT:** When giving an injection to a cat, slide the animal slowly across the top of the table. In most cases the cat will be concentrating on maintaining its footing and will not be aware of the injection. Another method of distraction is to place the plastic cover from a disposable needle on the examination table near the patient. Just before the injection is to be given, roll the cover slowly in front of the animal.

* * * * * *

377. **BETTER BACKFLOW:** For intravenous injections in cats, use a 25-gauge, 3/8 in. needle. This gives a better back-flow of blood into a glass-tipped syringe than does the 26-gauge needle. (Ed. note: The use of a clear plastic-hubbed needle makes the back-flow even more visible.)

* * * * * *

378. **MINIMUM RESTRAINT:** To collect a small amount of blood from a cat, clamp a stout rubber band above the elbow with a hemostat. Without attaching a syringe, insert a 25-gauge needle into the vein and allow the hub to fill. The hub contains enough blood for a few blood smears and for determining packed cell volume. The advantage of this procedure is that it requires little or no restraint and causes minimal excitement.

* * * * * *

379. **UROLITHIASIS:** When treating urolithiasis in male cats, use a 23-gauge, Luer-Slip, straight lacrimal needle to flush the penis.

* * * * * *

380. **MINIMIZE TRAUMA:** To unblock and flush the urethra in a cat, use an Abbocath-T® (Abbott) radiopaque intravenous catheter. This Teflon, 20 gauge × 1½ inch catheter causes very little trauma.

381. **DECREASE NEPHROTOXITY:** When unplugging a cat, give 0.5 to 1 cc of Psymod™ (Pitman-Moore) with atropine intravenously. This combination is less nephrotoxic to cats than other anesthetics.

******

382. **INDUCE URINE FLOW:** When treating a male cat with urolithiasis and a complete obstruction, use Cetacaine® (Haver-Lockhart) for treatment. The tip of the applicator is gently inserted into the distal end of the penis and a quick spray is administered. This results in a flushing effect, producing an immediate flow of urine.

******

383. **ASPIRATE THE URINE:** When treating an acute urethral obstruction in the cat, attach the end of the catheter to a suction pump and aspirate the urine. This helps draw out sediment that might remain in the bladder. After suctioning is complete, flush the bladder with sterile saline solution and repeat the suction procedure. The catheter is then left in the cat for two days.

******

384. **USEFUL NEEDLES:** Probe pointed needles, Vita Needle Company, Needham, Mass. — 22, 20, 18, 16, and 14 ga. have many uses. Urethral impactions, blockages of the naso-lacrimal ducts, anal gland injections, etc. One inch usually is enough. Keep a supply on hand — sterile — in test tubes and cotton.

******

385. **HEAT CATHETER:** When leaving an in-dwelling plastic or polyethylene catheter in a cat, use a lighted match to heat the exposed end and form a flange so the catheter will not work its way up into the bladder.

******

386. **FLUSHING MIXTURE:** An excellent preparation for flushing the bladder of a "plugged-up" tom cat is a mixture of Furacin® solution (Norden), vinegar and DMSO. To increase bladder tone, use a combination of Urecholine® (Merck) and ampicillin or Garamycin® (Schering).

****

387. **REDUCE BLEEDING:** In treatment of feline hemorrhagic urolithiasis, Lasix® (National) reduces bleeding significantly. The dose for the average cat is 0.5 to 1 cc. The Lasix® may be given alone or mixed with intravenous fluids.

******

388. **SUTURE CATHETER:** In obstinate cases of urethral obstruction in male cats, insert a tom cat catheter and suture it into place so that it can be retained for one or two days. Keep the cat on a slatted floor to prevent it from becoming soiled with dribbling urine.

******

389. **PREVENT UROLITHIASIS:** To prevent urinary urolithiasis in cats, increase water intake by adding extra salt (500 mg/kg of body weight). Add one teaspoonful per pound of canned food.

******

390. **URECHOLINE®** (Merck) is the best drug for overcoming "bladder wall exhaustion".

******

391. **MANY PLUGGED CATS** have negative urine cultures and struvite crystals without clinical infection.

******

392. **LOWER PH:** To lower the urine pH in cats, give pediatric vitamin C drops daily and feed Prescription Diet c/d® (Hill). Prescription Diet c/d® shifts urine to the acid side.

******

393. **MINERALS AFFECT FUS:** Cats with FUS (feline urological syndrome) are benefited by diets low in phosphorus and magnesium.

******

394. **ENCOURAGE WATER CONSUMPTION:** Always make a large dish of fresh water available to a cat being treated for cystitis.

******

395. **TASTY MEDICATION:** Some feline medications can be administered by adding the material to clam juice.

******

396. **PH VARIES:** Urine pH varies considerably during a 24 hour period. Beware of too much reliance on one sample.

******

397. **CLEAN LITTER VITAL:** Dirty litter may initiate a urine retention habit. A vicious cycle is put in motion; alkaline urine, bacterial growth, crystals form, blockage, TROUBLE!!!

******

398. **ESTIMATING AGE:** A rule of thumb for estimating the age of young

kittens of either sex is to attribute 1 month of age to each pound of body weight—(up to 4½ months of age).

******

399. **INEXPENSIVE LITTER TRAYS:** Kaiser Aluminum rigid foil containers (10012) are just the right size (12½ in. long × 8 in. wide × 2 in. deep) for use as litter trays in cat cages. They may be used over and over again before they are discarded. They can also be used for storing dirty syringes, for disinfecting solutions, etc.. The trays are available in cartons of 250 from local paper supply houses at a cost of approximately 10 cents each.

******

400. **INEXPENSIVE LITTER:** All-Dry® is an inexpensive litter material available at most automotive supply stores.

******

401. **INSULATOR:** An excellent insulator for maintaining body heat following shock is the square Fro-gen® (Jen-Sal) styrofoam box used as a shipping container for biologics. Cut a hole in one end of the box so that the patient's head can protrude. The container is large enough to accommodate the body of a cat without leaving an excess of dead air space. The container is also a great insulated carrier for hot or cold foods.

******

402. **EASES BATHING:** When bathing and/or dipping a cat, place a piece of wire screen against the wall and allow one end to extend to the bottom of the tub. Place the cat on the screen and his claws will instinctively grab into the screen, allowing the cat to be bathed and dipped with fewer problems.

******

403. **PREPPING FOR SURGERY:** When prepping a cat for surgery, especially a long-haired cat, soap the area to a good lather and use a sharp Weck blade to shave the area. This eliminates the loose hair.

******

404. **REDUCE POISONING:** To prevent feline poisoning and possible death, write "For Dogs Only" on the labels of products you dispense for canine patients. This is especially important in the case of dips that a client might be tempted to apply to a cat.

******

405. **ALTERNATIVE MITICIDE:** In treatment of ear mites in cats, mix 2 cc of an undiluted benzene hexachloride pine oil tick dip, Hexrin®, with 250 cc of an injectable mastitis-type ointment and instill several drops into the ears with a disposable syringe.

* * * * * *

406. **DON'T FORGET THE TAIL:** When advising clients on the treatment of ear mites in cats, tell them to apply some of the medication to the end of the tail or to wipe any medication left on their fingers onto the tail. Cats sleep with the end of the tail curled next to the ears and mites may get on the tail and reinfest the ears if treatment of the tail is neglected.

* * * * * *

407. **ANTISERUM FOR EXPOSED CATS:** When kittens have been exposed to distemper, vaccinate with homologous serum at a dose of 1 cc/lb. Order from Fromm Labs.

* * * * * *

408. **TOXEMIA:** Kittens will eat the common house plant dieffenbachia (Dumb Cane) resulting in signs of toxemia, often including loss of coordination. Recovery usually occurs spontaneously within eight to ten hours.

* * * * * *

409. **INTUBATION SAVES LIVES:** In cases of diaphragmatic hernia in cats, a considerable degree of atelectasis may be present as a result of pressure from the abdominal viscera. Many cats can be saved by tracheal intubation followed immediately by inflation of the lungs with gentle bag pressure.

* * * * * *

410. **APPETITE STIMULANT:** When a cat won't eat, try giving it 1 or 2 drops twice daily of the following mixture: 1 oz V.A.L.® Syrup (Fort Dodge) plus 2 cc Predef 2X® (Upjohn).

* * * * * *

411. **DON'T CAUTERIZE ULCERS:** In cats, mild corneal ulcers without secondary vascularization heal through a remodeling of existing cells rather than growth of new cells. Cautery dehydrates existing cells, reducing their ability to engage in the remodeling process.

* * * * * *

412. **FLUSH DUCTS:** In cats with conjunctivitis, the lacrimal ducts should be flushed with sterile saline solution. PE 20 intradermic polyethylene

tubing fitted with a 26-27 gauge needle is excellent for this purpose.

* * * * * *

413. **REDUCES SALAVATION:** Atropine ophthalmic ointment produces less slobbering in cats than does atropine drops.

* * * * * *

414. **INHALATION THERAPY:** Improve recovery in cases of feline rhinotracheitis by providing aerosol therapy and maintaining nutritional intake through the use of a pharyngostomy tube. For aerosol therapy, cover a cage with cardboard and cut out a window. Spray Mucomyst® (Mead Johnson) into the cage through a garden type sprayer for 15 minutes, three times daily.

* * * * * *

415. **SUPPORTIVE THERAPY:** In treatment of feline respiratory diseases always consider the use of parenteral fluids as supportive therapy.

* * * * * *

416. **EXPECTORANT FOR CATS:** Use a vaporizer containing 100,000 units of pancreatic dornase, Dornavac® (Merck), and 100,000 units of penicillin in 8 oz of water.

* * * * * *

417. **VITAMIN C:** Give 500 mg of vitamin C in a.m. and p.m. for treatment of feline respiratory viral infections.

* * * * * *

418. **ULTRAVIOLET LIGHTS:** Prevent spread of feline viral infections by installing 50% more ultraviolet lights than recommended. Keep bulbs free from dust. Do not allow rays to contact eyes.

* * * * * *

419. **IMPROVE SENSE OF SMELL:** Chlorpheniramine, Telodron® (Norden) in sustained-release form was used successfully to treat 45 of 55 cats with moderate to severe signs of FVR (feline viral rhinotracheitis). Favorable response was attributed to the prompt drying effect produced by chlorpheniramine in clearing nasal passages and improving sense of smell. This helped to reduce anorexia and subsequent mortality. Results were favorable with chlorpheniramine alone and in combination with antibiotics. Treatment of previous cases with antibiotics alone had been unsuccessful.

* * * * * *

420. **TRIPLE PLAY:** Cats require three times the dose of corticosteroids given to dogs.

******

421. **NUISANCE SPRAYING:** Administer 100 mg medroxyprogesterone, Deep-Provera® (Upjohn) intramuscularly or subcutaneously for a full grown entire or castrated male or 50-100 mg for an adult spayed female (not recommended for unspayed females). Repeat if necessary.

******

422. **GRISIOFULVIN DOSAGE FOR CATS:**
   A. Give with fat to increase absorption.
   B. Mix with fish and oil.
   C. 30 mg/lb/day.
   D. Always give after meal.
   E. Give Weladol™ (Pitman-Moore) bath to control hair infection.
   F. Clean up area.

******

423. **HAIR BALL TREATMENT:** Methyl cellulose, Mucilose® (Winthrop) is a good treatment for hair balls in cats.

******

424. **HAIR BALL PREVENTION:** To prevent hair balls in cats, recommend the daily addition of ½ teaspoon of cooking oil to the cat's food.

******

425. **CHEMOTHERAPY FOR FIP CASES:** Over the past few years a number of treatments have been advocated for FIP (feline infectious peritonitis). By the time many cats are brought to the veterinarian, the disease is advanced, organ damage is substantial, and the animals are anorectic and very debilitated. These cats are extremely poor candidates for treatment and should probably be euthanatized. If the cat is still in good flesh, the appetite is still good, and severe organ damage has not occurred, treatment can be considered if the owner desires. Co-infection with FELV (feline leukemia virus), occuring in about one-half of the cases of FIP, does not necessarily preclude treatment, especially if there are no other symptoms of FELV related disease (bone marrow dyscrasias, other secondary infections, neoplasia). The most effective treatment consists of immuno-suppressive and anti-inflammatory drugs coupled with good supportive care. Prednisolone or prednisone, 1½ to 2 mg/lb/day, and cyclophosphamide, 1 mg/lb daily for 4 consecutive days of each week, are beneficial when used in combination.

Phenylalanine mustard, Alkeran®, 2-2½ mg tablets, ¼ tablet every other day can be substituted for the cyclophosphamide. Treatment is continued for as long as progressive improvement is seen. Failure to produce improvement in several weeks, or deterioration of condition, are indications of treatment failure. Drug therapy is reinstituted if clinical symptoms return or if the serum antibody titer begins to rise. This type of therapy is effective in inducing remissions in about one-third of the cases presented. Unfortunately, many of these cats will have a relapse.

* * * * * *

426. **INAPPROPRIATE DEFECATION:** Some cats will defecate outside the litter pan even though otherwise house trained. In the absence of other physical disease, emotional trauma or unclean litter, express the anal sacs. Pressure from impacted anal sacs may cause inconsistent defecation. If impacted anal sacs are expressed, many otherwise healthy cats will resume normal defecatory habits the same day.

* * * * * *

427. **REMOVE ODORS:** V-Tergent™ (Pitman-Moore) is an effective product for removing the odor and oils associated with stud tail in male cats. Wash as necessary to control condition and remove sebum.

* * * * * *

428. **URINE ODOR:** To neutralize cat urine, wash with V-Tergent™ or a similar product and rinse with vinegar and water.

* * * * * *

429. **PERSIANS** commonly have ringworm. Always check kittens under a Wood's lamp.

* * * * * *

430. **BIRTH DEFECTS:** Never give grisiofulvin to pregnant queens. It may cause birth defects.

* * * * * *

431. **MAY CAUSE PNEUMONIA:** Toxoplasmosis may cause acute pneumonia in kittens and cats. Test blood titers. Symptoms are hard and fast breathing and high temperature with no response to antibiotics. Try Tribressen® (Burroughs-Wellcome) for treatment.

* * * * * *

432. **DIRECT SMEAR:** Trichomonas causes soft stool/diarrhea. Diagnose by direct smear with saline. Treat with Flagyl® (Searle) 125 mg t.i.d., or Atabrine® (Winthrop) 25 mg b.i.d..

433. **BLOOD TO MUSCLE:** To diagnose trichinosis in cats fed raw meat, check the sediment of your flotation solution. Larvae spread in blood to muscle. Treat with thiabendazole (25 mg/lb).

* * * * * *

434. **ASPIRIN MAY BE TOXIC:** Aspirin in doses used for a dog is very toxic to cats. It may cause aplastic anemia. It can be used when indicated in smaller doses.

* * * * * *

435. **VITAMIN C HELPFUL:** Tylenol® (McNeil) is toxic to cats. It causes brown urine and bluish mucus membranes, hemolytic anemia, and liver damage. Vitamin C may be of some help.

* * * * * *

436. **TOXIC TO CATS:** Dipyrone is very toxic to cats. It may cause aplastic anemia.

* * * * * *

437. **ALCOHOL I.V.:** Oxalate poisoning in cats is caused by consuming anti-freeze, eating spinach, eating house plants such as philodendron or oxalis. Treat with intravenous ethyl alcohol.

* * * * * *

438. **HERBICIDES ARE TOXIC:** Cats are very susceptible to herbicides such as 2-4-D. It is toxic to the liver. There is no treatment and it is hard to diagnose.

* * * * * *

439. **ADENOCARCINOMA:** Siamese cats that have recurrent vomiting may have adenocarcinoma of the intestines.

* * * * * *

440. **THERAPY FOR RENAL FAILURE:** The following generalities are intended for use only as long as renal failure persists:
    A. Avoid "shotgun" therapy.
       1. Do not administer drugs to uremic cats unless there is a specific indication for their action.
       2. Antibiotics should not be given prophylactically. They are best reserved for use when there is evidence of infection. (They may be used prophylactically after renal failure has been corrected.)

* * * * * *

441. **HYPOCALCEMIA:** Kittens that are sore, have thin bones, and weak

legs often have hypocalcemia. Give calcium gluconate and change their diets. The patient will improve overnight.

******

442. **ENTHANASIA BY INTRAPERITONEAL INJECTION:** When a cat must be euthanatized, a method that is easy on the cat, the aide, the practitioner, and the client is intraperitoneal injection of a concentrated pentobarbital solution. The aide holds the cat by the scruff of the neck with one hand and with the other hand vigorously massages the cat's forehead. While supporting the cat's abdomen and pelvis with the left hand, inject the pentobarbital into the abdominal cavity from the right side, about in the center of the abdomen. The method allows the cat to be lightly restrained in a natural position (*i.e.* standing). The rubbing of the forehead seems to distract the cat while the injection is given.

******

443. **HOT BATH:** When neonates delivered by cesarean section are depressed, cold, and have irregular respiration, submerge them to the neck in a hot bath (103 degrees F) for several minutes. This effectively improves all three conditions simultaneously.

******

444. **ISOLETTE PROVIDES CONTROLLED ENVIRONMENT:** An Isolette provides controlled temperature environment for orphan pups and a place to keep puppies until the dam is awake from cesarean section. A used Isolette unit can often be purchased from a hospital supply house.

******

445. **HIP DYSPLASIA PREVENTION:** Dr. Wendell O. Belfield, San Jose, California, has found he could completely prevent hip dysplasia in puppies from dysplastic parents by feeding ascorbate. The regimen recommended is as follows: 2 to 4 grams of sodium ascorbate in the daily ration of the pregnant bitch. At birth the pups are given 50 to 100 mg of Ce-Vi-Sol® (Mead Johnson) by mouth. When pups are 3 weeks of age, Ce-Vi-Sol® is replaced by 500 mg of sodium ascorbate daily until the pups are 4 months old. The dosage is then increased to 1 to 2 grams daily and continued until the pups are 18 to 24 months of age.

******

446. **FECAL IMPACTIONS:** Innovar-Vet™ (Pitman-Moore) injection given intravenously is useful in manually breaking down "concrete" fecal im-

91

pactions in dogs. The analgesia and sedation produced allows you to break down fecal masses with forceps and to administer softening solution with minimal discomfort to the patient.

******

447. **HYGOCLYCEMIA RESULT OF STRESS:** Young puppies that have been subject to the stress of shipment usually exhibit hypoglycemia. The condition can be successfully treated with 1 to 2 cc of 50% dextrose given intravenously.

******

448. **BARIUM ENEMA:** For conveneince in administering a barium enema to small animals, fill a 4½ oz disposable enema bottle with a barium solution. Prior to taking the radiograph, insert the nozzle into the rectum and expel the barium solution into the previously emptied colon.

******

449. **FISH HOOK REMOVAL:** For easy removal of a fish hook from the esophagus of a dog, first offer the animal bread. Then give an intravenous injection of xylazine, Rompun® (Haver-Lockhart), at a dosage of 0.5 cc/20 lb body weight, in conjunction with an appropriate dose of atropine sulfate. In most cases, vomiting occurs within 60 seconds, producing the fish hook.

******

450. **DOWNWARD PRESSURE:** To remove a fish hook that is not too deeply inbedded, apply downward pressure on the eye of the hook and then pull back quickly on the curve of the needle.

******

451. **FEED BREAD:** When a dog has chewed and swallowed foreign matter (such as a plastic toy), force feed some bread before administering an emetic.

******

452. **LESION EASILY OBSERVED:** The plastic case from a disposable syringe is an effective bandage for protecting the tip of the tail. Slip the plastic case, open at both ends, over the injury and tape it in place at the cranial end. The lesion can be easily observed through the clear plastic case.

******

453. **HYPERVENTILATION:** In cases of hyperventilation in dogs (be sure to differentiate from heat exhaustion), administer a tranquilizer and

place the dog's head in a paper bag to increase the level of carbon dioxide.

* * * * * *

454. **CANINE ARTIFICIAL RESPIRATION:** When giving artificial respiration to a dog, first check for a patent airway. With the dog in lateral recumbency, press down firmly over the rib cage to expel the air. Then grasp a large fold of skin over the ribs (two hands may be required if the dog is large) and pull until the animal is almost lifted from the table. The sound of air being taken in is usually audible. The cycle is repeated as necessary. A dog can be kept alive with this procedure until supplemental oxygen is available.

* * * * * *

455. **FOOT TOUGHENER:** An effective homemade foot-toughener for hunting dogs is a mixture of 30 cc tincture of benzoin, 1 oz alum, 2 oz tannic acid, 8 oz petroleum jelly, and 10 cc balsam of peru. Apply the mixture daily.

* * * * * *

456. **CLOROX® REMOVES PLASTER:** Traces of casting plaster may be removed easily with a Clorox® solution. The acid solution converts the insoluble plaster carbonates that adhere to the hands and instruments into soluble chlorides that rinse away rapidly with tap water. If the solution is used to dissolve traces of plaster clinging to the patients coat, care must be taken to prevent the solution from contacting and dissolving the freshly-applied cast.

* * * * * *

457. **CATSUP INCREASES PALATABILITY:** For dogs that won't eat food with Styrid-Caricide® (American Cyanamid) added, mix catsup with the ration and spread additional catsup over the top. Several of my clients told me about this, and it works.

* * * * * *

458. **PREVENT ACUTE GASTRIC DILATATION:** Moistening dry dog food 30 minutes before feeding may aid in preventing acute gastric dilatation.

* * * * * *

459. **DEPRAVED APPETITE:** Treat pica in young dogs with a combination of Viokase® (Robins) and lixotinic. The depraved appetite (for wood, dirt, grass, feces, stones) may be the result of a vitamin-mineral deficiency. This deficiency occurs in young dogs that are teething and experiencing faulty digestion of food.

460. **ACUTE UREMIC EPISODES:** A number of cases have been reported of older dogs developing acute uremic episodes when fed only meat.

******

461. **POOR DEVELOPMENT:** A dark, foul-smelling diarrhea may be developed by weanling puppies being fed "all meat" foods. The diarrhea is accompanied by weight reductions and loss of condition of musculature and hair coat. The condition is unresponsive to usual antibiotic and supportive therapy. Cessation of "all meat" foods, however, results in dramatic and rapid resumption of normal bowel movements, regaining of weight, and the restoration of hair coat and muscle condition. Nutritional secondary hyperparathyroidism is a calcium deficiency that can occur in growing dogs and cats being fed exclusively "all meat" foods.

******

462. **ANTIBODIES ARE PROTEIN:** When an animal is undernourished, some theorize that the body utilizes antibody proteins to meet its demand for protein, reducing the animal's immunity to infectious agents. A formula for orphan puppies is ¼ pint light cream; ¾ pint homogenized milk; 1 egg yolk.
When hunting dogs are worked, feed them ¼ of a day's ration two hours before they go into the field. Feed the remainder at the end of the day after the hunting is finished.

******

463. **HALITOSIS:** Halitosis in Spaniels is often caused by lip-fold pyoderma. This area should be removed surgically and sutured with stainless steel wire. Other causes of halitosis are bad teeth, tonsillitis, and chronic esophagitis. In treating the latter condition, a low-level antibiotic powder such as Entromycin™ (Pitman-Moore) may be of value.

******

464. **LOW CALCIUM BRINGS RELIEF:** A mild arthritic condition can be relieved by supplying half the ration as lean meat and the other half with a proprietary dog food and water. The lower calcium content is probably the source of relief.

******

465. **USE CORN OIL:** Mild diabetes or sugar in the urine can often be cleared by reducing the amount of proprietary food and supplementing it with corn oil as a source of calories.

******

466. **COPPER DEFICIENCY:** Animals fed a diet entirely of meat may develop anemia from copper deficiency. This often changes the color and texture of the hair..

******

467. **DECREASE IN SENSE OF SMELL:** Anemia in bird dogs may cause a decrease in smelling ability (Hb. below 8 gm). Raw liver helps.

******

468. **EAR WASH:** An effective ear wash for smelly ears can be made by mixing 1 teaspoon of V-Tergent 8X™ (Pitman-Moore) with 1 cup of water.

******

469. **ANTIBIOTICS 'DU JOUR':** A majority of ear problems need only air. Remove hair, locally and as needed. Wash the ear once or twice a day, or twice a week as needed. Use 1 or 2 tablespoons of white vinegar and a glass of warm water. Pour in ear and let dog shake its head. Antibiotics 'du jour". A dog that needs a La Croiux procedure can benefit by having the ears taped over it's head for 3 to 4 weeks, postoperative.

******

470. **HAIR REMOVAL:** Remove hair from the ear canal in a poodle by applying Surgex® and then syringe out the ear. This facilitates the removal of debris and creates a healthier area.

******

471. **REMOVAL OF WAX AND DEBRIS:** For rapid removal of wax and debris from the ear canal of a dog or cat, fill the ear with Surfak® (Hoechst) enema solution. The solution does not burn or irritate raw tissue and it leaves the ear clean and free of grease. The solution appears to be compatible with most other medications.

******

472. **A BASIC PREPARATION FOR EAR INFECTIONS:**
8 oz tannic acid, U.S.P.
4 oz boric acid, U.S.P.
2 oz salicylic acid, U.S.P., fine crystals
Put in clean gallon bottle and add 70% alcohol
Qs to make 1 gallon.

******

473. **EXCESSIVE WAX:** As an aid in treating chronic ear infection and otoacariasis complicated by the presence of excessive wax, use Debrox® (International Pharmaceutical Corp.) to rid the ears of wax. The pro-

duct can be purchased at any drug store and may be used indefinitely.

******

474. **PH AIDS THERAPY:** In treating otitis, the pH of ear exudate can serve as a guide to therapy. Use Nitrazine® paper (Squibb) to determine the pH. If the specimen is acid, treat for allergy; if the specimen is alkaline, treat for bacterial infection.

******

475. **SEBORRHEA:** Ear margin crusting is often due to seborrhea or scabies. Ear notch (tip) infections should be removed surgically or taped to the head for ten days. Apply steroid ointment daily.

******

476. **ADD 5% VINEGAR** to Furacin® (Norden) solution you dispense for ear problems.

******

477. **CHRONIC OTITIS:** An excellent preparation for treating recurrent and chronic otitis is VoSol® drops (Wallace). This product contains 1-2 propanediol diacetate 3%, acetate acid 2%, benzethonium chloride 0.02%, propylene glycol, and hydrocortisone 1%. It offers wide antibacterial, antifungal, antiinflammatory, and antipruritic activity.

******

478. **RESISTANT CHRONIC OTITIS** may involve a fungal infection. Such cases often respond to oral administration of griseofulvin, Fulvicin® (Schering).

******

479. **BITE REPELLENT:** A repellent for fly bites on the ears and nose of a dog: oil of citronella, 1 part; mineral oil, 10 parts. Dab on the affected areas.

******

480. **TICK REMOVAL:** Remove individual ticks from a dog by using a medicine dropper. Place several drops of the bovine grubicide, Warbex® (American Cyanamid), directly on the body of the tick.

******

481. **TREATING CONCHAL HEMATOMA:** After the hematoma is organized, incise it and inject 1 mg of Azium® (Schering). To provide drainage, suture a Larson's teat canula in the ear. Leave the canula in the ear for about two weeks.

******

482. **EAR MITES AFFECT PERFORMANCE:** There is evidence that ear mite infection may cause Beagles to stop barking while trailing a rabbit. Dogs brought to the veterinarian with this complaint invariably are infested with ear mites. Dipping the dog and treating the ears usually permits the dog to perform satisfactorily.

****

483. **EAR FLUSH:** Add 10 cc's of Weladol™ (Pitman-Moore) disinfectant to 4 ounces of hydrogen peroxide to flush out chronic infections, etc. Use in a plastic squeeze bottle with a tip.

******

484. **ANAL ADENOMA:** To treat anal adenomas in dogs that are poor surgical risks, inject 0.5 to 1 cc of diethylstilbestrol directly into the adenoma. Large adenomas may require three to four injections at weekly intervals.

******

485. **OPTIMAL DOSAGE:** Drs. Roger Yeary and Richard Brant, Ohio State University, have determined that the optimal dosage of aspirin for the dog is 25 to 35 mg per kg of body weight every 8 hours. For example, the dosage for a 30 lb dog would be one-half of a 5 grain aspirin every 8 hours.

******

486. **SUPPLEMENTAL ZINC:** Demodectic mange in dogs can be cured or arrested by feeding supplemental zinc. The condition often recurs when the treatment is stopped.

******

487. **TOOTHPASTE:** 10% Weladol™ makes a good toothpaste for dogs with bad breath. You won't have to ask where the yellow went.

******

488. **INEXPENSIVE DOSE SYRINGE:** A kitchen baster, available in the housewares section of department stores, makes an inexpensive dose syringe for administering large doses of liquid drugs.

******

489. **VERSATILE CANNULAS:** An udder infusion cannula with a Luer hub can be autoclaved and used for artificial insemination in canine practice. These cannulas are also useful for flushing wounds and, connected to a vacuum apparatus or hypodermic syringe, for aspirating fluids.

490. **ARTIFICIAL INSEMINATION:** A device for introducing semen into a bitch is a Becton-Dickinson laryngeal cannula. This cannula can be autoclaved and it fits directly onto a syringe.

* * * * * *

491. **BALLING GUN:** To administer capsules, boluses, or tablets to small animals that are difficult to handle, cut the end from a disposable syringe and use the syringe as a balling gun.

* * * * * *

492. **DISTRACT DOG:** To keep a dog distracted while giving it an injection, smear a small amount of peanut butter on the roof of the dog's mouth before inserting the needle. For cats, substitute Nutri-Cal® (EVSCO) for the peanut butter. This simple step keeps the patient preoccupied while the injection is being given.

* * * * * *

493. **LUBRICATE CAPSULES:** When giving large capsules to dogs, coat the capsule with a small amount of K-Y® lubricating jelly.

* * * * * *

494. **TISSUE PAPER:** To give several small tablets at the same time, wrap them in a small piece of tissue paper and administer as you would a single large tablet.

* * * * * *

495. **INEXPENSIVE COVERS:** The plastic lids provided with many products packaged in cans (Pringles's Potato Chips®, Hershey's Chocolate Syrup®, tennis balls, etc.) make excellent covers for opened and unused cans of dog food.

* * * * * * *

496. **PROTECTION:** Vinyl disposable gloves protect not only the patient but the doctor. Use them when tattooing, applying iodine, methylene blue, or any other preparation where staining may be a problem.

* * * * * *

497. **RECYCLE DISPOSABLES:** If you encounter shortages of plastic items and disposables, try washing and autoclaving them. Most of these items will stand up well under this "recycling".

* * * * * *

498. **FLEA SPRAY REMOVES STAINS:** To remove gentian violet or pyocyanin blue stains from the hands, spray the stained areas with flea spray before washing.

499. **BLOOD STAIN REMOVAL:** To eliminate blood stains on patients' coats, keep a pint bottle of hydrogen peroxide with a Windex® sprayer attached in the surgery and treatment rooms. Spray areas of hemorrhage as needed.

* * * * * *

500. **SKUNK ODOR:** To deodorize a dog that has come in contact with a skunk, bathe the animal in Micrin® mouth wash.

* * * * * *

501. **IODINE REMOVES STAINS:** To remove silver nitrate stains from the skin and objects, apply an iodine preparation. The iodine can be rinsed off later with alcohol, soap and water.

* * * * * *

502. **GO-JO REMOVES TAR:** When an animal is brought in coated with heavy oil of the type used to hold down road dust and prepare roads for asphalt surfacing, apply an opthalmic ointment to the eyes and clean the entire body with a mechanics waterless handcleaner (*e.g.* Go-jo). After a thorough application and rubbing, wash the cleaner and oil off with a good shampoo. Repeat as necessary.

* * * * * *

503. **TAR REMOVAL:** Mineral oil is a safe and effective solvent for removing tar from the coat of animals.

* * * * * *

504. **REDUCE ODOR:** To reduce the odor of dips such as ronnel, add 2 capfuls of Sanzyme® (Summit Hill) concentrate (odor neutralizer) with 1 ml. of lemon citrus oil concentrate (available at novelty shops) to the dip solution.

* * * * * *

505. **PREWARM SOLUTIONS:** To have prewarmed sterile saline solution always ready for flushing abdominal or throatic cavities, keep the solution in a laboratory incubator at 37^0 C. Intravenous fluids can be prewarmed in the same way.

* * * * * *

506. **KEEP BEVEL UPWARD:** When giving intravenous injections, be sure the bevel of the needle is up. When the needle is threaded into the vein, exert slight upward pressure so the bevel will slide along the top of the vein.

* * * * * *

507. **USE EAR FOR VENIPUNCTURE:** Venipuncture in achondroplastic dogs, such as the Basset and Dachshund, can be simplified by swabbing the exterior of the ear with alcohol. This makes the veins clearly visible. Use a 20 or 22-ga. needle. Since this procedure seems to cause little pain, minimal restraint is required.

******

508. **CROOKED CEPHALIC VEINS:** For venipunctures in a Dachshund or Basset hound with crooked cephalic veins, use a 23-ga., ¾ inch Yale® disposable needle. Insert it into one of the readily accessible auricular veins.

******

509. **INJECT INTO LUMBAR MUSCLE:** Use lumbar muscle area for intramuscular injections in dogs and cats. Avoid using the thigh muscles for intramuscular injections to minimize the owner's complaint that the injection caused lameness in the dog. Use fine gauge short needle.

******

510. **FLEX TO REDUCE PAIN:** Flexing the hind limb relaxes the muscles and allows a less painful intramuscular administration of either vaccines or therapeutic agents.

******

511. **TRANQUILIZERS INCREASE APPETITE:** Tranquilizers occasionally make excellent appetite stimulants for homesick dogs and cats that will not eat while hospitalized or boarded.

******

512. **MAKESHIFT HOT WATER BOTTLE:** If a hot water bottle is not available, fill surgical gloves with hot water and close the ends tightly with a rubber band.

******

513. **EMERGENCY KITS:** In those situations where seconds count, emergency kits (containing a sterile disposable syringe, Adrenalin® (Parke, Davis), antihistamine, etc.) strategically placed about the hospital can be life savers.

******

514. **CHRONIC DIARRHEA IN DOGS:** Use 1 level teaspoon of Tylan ® (Elanco) in food b.i.d..

******

515. **STEROID ENEMA:** When treating recurring episodes of severe colitis,

in addition to administering daily medication, have the patient returned monthly as necessary for a steroid enema. Depo-Medrol® (Upjohn), given under sedation via a retention enema and mixed with Kaopectate® (Upjohn), is often beneficial.

* * * * * *

516. **VOMITING AND DIARRHEA TREATMENT:** Add 1 package (45 gm.) of Sulkamycin-S® powder (Norden) to 3 oz. of hot water in a blender or high-speed mixer. While mixing, slowly add 13 oz. of warmed Karo® syrup. Continue mixing until the suspension is consistent. Store in the refrigerator. Dispense in 2-oz. dropper bottles and give at the rate of 1 teaspoon (5 cc.) every six hours until the vomiting and/or diarrhea stops.

* * * * * *

517. **BE PREPARED:** To save precious seconds in emergency situations, keep emergency parenteral solutions (epinephrine, nalorphine, anesthetic antagonists, etc.) in sterile syringes. Clearly label these solutions with a marking pen.

* * * * * *

518. **ADMINISTER EARLY AND FREQUENTLY:** When using antimicrobial agents, administer large doses early and frequently — then stop. Do not attempt to build dosage levels or to taper off the dosage.

* * * * * *

519. **DIGESTION AID:** To break down the starch cells and minimize coprophagy, soak dry commercial dog food with very hot water.

* * * * * *

520. **COPROPHAGY:** To reduce coprophagy, give glutamic acid orally in capsule form.

* * * * * *

521. **ADOLPH'S AIDS DIGESTION:** To minimize coprophagy and flatulence in dogs, sprinkle Adolph's Meat Tenderizer® on the dog's food each day.

* * * * * *

522. **OVER-EATING:** Highly palatable pet foods may be overconsumed.

* * * * * *

523. **KEEP IN MIND:** Overweight pet owners have overweight pets.

* * * * * *

524. **OBESITY** adds to pain when sick or injured.

******

525. **FLUID REPLACEMENT:** To compensate for loss of water, electrolytes and bicarbonate caused by diarrhea, give Lactated Ringer's solution. To compensate for loss of water, electrolytes and chloride resulting from vomiting, give 2½ % dextrose in a half-strength saline solution.

******

526. **CLEANING AND DISINFECTING:** To clear up diarrheal enteritis, use a combination of Tide® and Clorox® as a cleaning and disinfecting solution. Use 1 cup of Tide® and 1 cup of Clorox® in water to clean the runs and cages once daily until the problem has been eliminated. Then use the solution once a week. Within one month the diarrhea problem should disappear.

******

527. **DONNATAL® FOR BOXERS:** Donnatal® (Robins) will help Boxers that eat grass and vomit.

******

528. **FEED GELFOAM®** (Upjohn) in severe cases of gastrointestinal bleeding.

******

529. **CHRONIC GASEOUS DIARRHEA:** Atabrine® (Winthrop) tablets, 100mg., administered for four days may help some chronic gaseous diarrheas. Skip 4 days and repeat if needed. Do not exceed 100 mg./day — small dogs ¼ to ½ tablet.

******

530. **PECTIN USEFUL FOR LOOSE STOOLS:** In order to regulate a loose stool, thoroughly mix equal parts of canned stewed tomatoes, rice and hamburger. The pectin in the tomato pulp apparently aids in the digestion and transportation of the residue. This diet is an excellent adjunct to enteritis therapy. Vitamin and mineral supplementation is necessary with long-term use.

******

531. **GASTRIC DILATATION:** To prevent gastric dilatation in large dogs, instruct the owners to feed the dog three or four small meals daily instead of one or two large meals. This schedule does not allow a large amount of easily digestible carbohydrates to accumulate in the stomach. The dog should also be prevented form exercising vigorously for at

least two or three hours after eating.

******

532. **SALT AS AN EMETIC:** Whole table salt is an excellent emetic given orally. The dosage for dogs is 1 tablespoon; for cats, 1 teaspoon. Emesis usually occurs in one to five minutes.

******

533. **NAUSEA AND VOMITING:** When resuming alimentary feeding, after an episode of nausea or vomiting in a dog, give a mixture of equal parts of orange juice and Karo® syrup. The effective dosage is 1 to 3 teaspoons every one to two hours for twelve to twenty-four hours before water and solid food are offered.

******

534. **WINNING COMBINATIONS:** An excellent antiemetic-antidiarrheal injection is a combination of Tigan® (Beecham) and Centrine® (Bristol). These two drugs seem to mix well and do not create adverse reaction or toxicity.

******

535. **MAINTAIN POTASSIUM LEVEL:** Signs of polydypsia, polyuria, muscle fatigue, and generalized weakness which often follow injection of corticosteroids can be minimized by giving the patient foods that are rich in potassium. Cortisone therapy increases the retention of sodium and excretion of potassium. Sodium retention results in polydypsia and ensuing polyuria, while loss of potassium causes generalized weakness and muscle fatigue. Foods that contain a large amount of potassium are: powdered milk, bran flakes, molasses, fish, meat and fruit juices. When a client reports that a dog being treated with corticosteroids is drinking and urinating excessively, recommend that the animal be given Gatorade®, powdered milk, etc., rather than water.

******

536. **MISMATE:** When a female dog has been mismated and the client wants conception blocked, administer stilbestrol on the 5th to 7th day after the mating.

******

537. **POST-PARTUM TREATMENT FOR DOGS:** For an average 25-30 lb. bitch, give a tablet of 0.2 mg. per day of ergonovine for 5 days to prevent post-partum metritis.

******

538. **ECLAMPSIA:** When eclampsia in a bitch needs to be treated intravenously with no one to properly restrain the animal, give 15 gr./6 lb. body weight of chloral hydrate dissolved in 1 oz. water. The solution is given by rectal infusion with a Becton-Dickinson ear syringe (automatic plunger type with 1-in. attachment). Occasionally, a small additional dose may be needed. Isolate the bitch from her litter for 24 hours.

******

539. **HYPERVITAMINOSIS:** Pregnant bitches require 9 I.U.s of vitamin D per lb. of body weight per day. Dog breeders sometimes forget that many dog foods supply the required amount of vitamin D and supplement the diet of their breeding females with various forms of the vitamin. The result can be hypervitaminosis D. The lesions of overdosing with vitamin D are calcium deposits in the tongue and on the capsule of the liver in newborn pups.

******

540. **PROGESTERONE STIMULATES FIBROBLAST FORMATION:** Inject Depo Provera® (Upjohn) or repositol progesterone into hematoma, hygromas, capped hock, or shoe boil. Remove tissue fluid and inject the hormone.

******

541. **BONE MARROW RESPONSE:** Anabolic steroids may improve the bone marrow response in anemic and leucopenic animals not caused by cancer.

******

542. **OLD FEMALE DOGS** with chronic high urine pH, that are resistant to usual therapy, will respond to 1 mg. per day oral doses of stilbesterol.

******

543. **ODOR REMOVAL:** Bactine® (Miles) on corners where male dogs urinate will help eliminate odors.

******

544. **ECP® FOR RESISTANT INCONTINENCE:** ECP® (Upjohn), ½ to ¼ mg. is good for resistant incontinence in bitches. Larger doses of ECP® may produce aplastic anemia (as will estrogens). It takes up to 6 weeks to recover, if they live.

******

545. **TENDER LOVING CARE:** ECP® and estrogens will produce aplastic anemia. Many will recover if TLC is administered for six weeks.

* * * * * *

546. **MAST CELL TUMORS:** D.N.P.® (American Cyanamid) and steroids depress mast cell tumors better than either alone. 2 mg. Leukeran® (Burroughs Wellcome) per 30 lb. may help. Administer D.N.P.® at weekly intervals. Radiation therapy for 14 days after surgery is helpful.

* * * * * *

547. **URINARY INCONTINANCE** in male dogs may be relieved with 50 mg. Banthine® (Searle) t.i.d.

* * * * * *

548. **SPAY EARLY:** A dog will probably never get mammary tumors if she is spayed before her first heat. After four estrus cycles there will be no effect on occurrence of tumors. Also, indications are that spaying a dog with mammary tumors will not have an effect on the course of the disease.

* * * * * *

549. **ANABOLIC AGENTS AID RECOVERY:** After a long regimen of corticosteroid therapy, consider the use of an anabolic agent to assist the body's defense mechanism and to correct nitrogen imbalance.

* * * * * *

550. **DICOUMARIL POISONING:** Vitamin K^1 (human label) is the treatment of choice for dicoumaril poisoning. Vitamin K^3 is only 1/75th as effective a treatment as vitamin K^1.

* * * * * *

551. **HYPERTHYROIDISM:** The syndrome in nervous German Shepherds of intense itching and sweating may be hyperthyroidism. Try propylthiouracil, 100mg. t.i.d.

* * * * * *

552. **ENZYMES AND ULTRASOUND:** For treatment of herniated cervical and lumbar discs, give 1 proteolytic enzyme tablet Papase® (Warner-Chilcott) three times daily, and ultrasound. The ultrasonic treatment is given for three minutes daily for five days and then every other day until an additional five treatments have been administered. The dosage is 0.4 watts per CM². Treatment should begin as soon as possible. Muscle massage and exercise are also beneficial.

* * * * * *

553. **VITAMIN E AIDS OLD DOGS:** 200 mg. of vitamin E succinnate will act as an anabolic stimulant in older dogs that are thin.

* * * * * *

554. **CHRONIC NEPHRITICS:** Delatestryl® (Squibb) will aid chronic nephritis in older dogs with spinal problems. Give large breeds with flabby muscles in back legs 100 mg. every 3 weeks.

* * * * * *

555. **IN EMERGENCY SITUATIONS,** restore blood pressure quickly in a dog in shock by giving Canalb™ (Pitman-Moore) plasma protein solution as a rapid intravenous bolus. The method is safe and effective, and it gives the attending staff extra time to determine the cause of the shock.

* * * * * *

556. **CORTICOSTEROIDS FOR SHOCK:** Veterinarians should consider using massive doses of corticosteroids intravenously for shock. At least ten times the usual therapeutic dose should be administered intravenously to create the desired effect. The results are often dramatic in apparently terminal cases.

* * * * * *

557. **BALANCED NUTRITIONAL SUPPLEMENT:** An excellent preparation for providing a balanced nutritional supplement in the form of a parenteral solution is AA-1000® (Beecham). It can be given by any parenteral route in conjunction with fluid therapy. AA-1000® contains the 10 essential amino acids, B vitamins and electrolytes.

* * * * * *

558. **DEXAMETHASONE GIVEN I.V.** for shock must be acted on by the liver before it can act at the tissue level. Be sure to use intravenously those steroids that are in the succinate (soluble) form such as Solu-Delta-Cortef® (Upjohn).

* * * * * *

559. **TECHNIQUE FOR CONTROL OF INTRA-ABDOMINAL HEMORRHAGE:** A 4 ml. ampule of Levophed® (Winthrop) containing 4 mg. of levarterenol bitartrate is diluted to 100 to 200 ml. with 5% dextrose in water. The dosage ranges from 2-8 mg. of norepinephrine in 40-50 ml. of the fluid, depending on size of the animal. The diluted solution is administered intraperitoneally at a rapid rate. The animal is rolled gently and then placed in right lateral recumbency, especially if the liver is the suspected site of hemorrhage.

* * * * * *

560. **CONTROL OF LIVER AND PANCREATIC HEMORRHAGE:** Apply Surgicel® (Johnson & Johnson), an absorbable hemostatic, on sites of oozing hemorrhage to achieve hemostasis. It has wide application and can be used to successfully control hemorrhage of the liver and pancreas.

******

561. **VITAMIN C REDUCES INSULIN DOSAGE:** In treatment of diabetes in the dog, the daily dosage of insulin can be reduced several units by daily administration of 1 gm. of vitamin C.

******

562. **ACUTE PANCREATITIS:** When giving fluids, also give diurectic to prevent secondary pulmonary edema that often accompanies the condition.

******

563. **BICARBONATE:** Normally the pancreatic and bile ducts produce bicarbonate which helps to elevate the low pH (2.5-3) of stomach contents up to 7.5 or so. This basic pH is needed for chyme to function properly. In pancreatic disease, these ducts may produce insufficient quantities of bicarbonate.

******

564. **TOY DOGS THAT COLLAPSE** after vaccination will respond to intravenous glucose and/or Glucagon® (Lilly).

******

565. **REDUCE DOSAGE:** Greatly reduce the dosage of drugs when treating uremic dogs or cats. Such animals do not eliminate usual dosages of drugs. Only "distilled water" is eliminated by these animals. All other substances are filtered out and retained by the body. Under these circumstances, tetracyclines, neomycin, polymyxin, streptomycin, can be especially toxic.

******

566. **PRESCRIPTION DIETS** k/d® and u/d® (Hills) are low in minerals and protein. Dogs fed either diet produce low urine concentrations of calcium, phosphorus, magnesium, urates, and oxalates.

******

567. **GATORADE® FOR VOMITING:** Give Gatorade® to dogs that vomit water. Pour some over ice-cubes. Gatorade® supplies electrolytes that are lost in vomitus and dogs won't gulp it down as they do water.

******

107

568. **SEVEN MANIPULATIONS:** The azotemic dog with renal failure will benefit from 7 manipulations. It has been suggested that "Stabilize The Dog With Seven Vital Steps" may be used to remember this regimen of therapy with the following designations:
1. Stabilize — salt;
2. The — TLC, lack of stress;
3. Dog — diet;
4. With — water ad libitum;
5. Seven — sodium bicarbonate;
6. Vital — vitamins;
7. Steps — steroids, anabolic.

* * * * * *

569. **NOT ABSORBED:** Ringers or Lactated Ringers will be absorbed subcutaneously or intraperitoneally, whereas 5% dextrose will not. If given 5% dextrose intravenously, the dextrose is absorbed and metabolized and the extra water may produce a crisis such as in a pyometra-sick surgical patient.

* * * * * *

570. **AVOID SHOCK:** Treat abdominal ascites due to liver or cardiac pathology with a slow intravenous drip using Canalb™ (Pitman-Moore). By restoring colloid osmotic pressure, you may safely use diuresis or aspiration of fluid to treat ascitic patients and thus help avoid shock.

* * * * * *

571. **BABY SPOON:** To remove even the smallest calculi when performing a cystotomy, use a small baby spoon. The spoons are easy to sterilize.

* * * * * *

572. **COMMON DISEASE:** Pyelonephritis in dogs is more common than the diagnosed incidence indicates. Clinical signs may include varing degrees of some or all of the following: inappetance, fever, polydypsia, polyuria, vomiting, trembling, lethargy, and panting. Results of complete blood counts are usually within normal limits, especially in chronic cases. Urinalysis usually reveals proteinuria and cloudy urine. Specific gravity may be elevated in cases where there is a decrease in water consumption. The presence of tubular casts, pyuria, and bacteria in the stained urinary sediment usually confirms the diagnosis. Long-term antibiotic therapy is necessary and urine cultures are advisable. Untreated pyelonephritis may lead to chronic interstitial nephritis (end stage of renal disease).

573. **STONES VS. INFECTIONS:** Dogs with bladder stones have a high incidence of gram-positive (staph - strep) infections while dogs with uncomplicated cystitis have predominantly gram-negative infections. (coli-klebsiella-proteus-pseudomonas).

******

574. **HEMORRHAGE CONTROL:** One percent formalin rinse followed with a saline rinse is useful for severe hematuria. This procedure helps following removal of bladder stones in dogs and also helps control bleeding from dogs given Cytoxan® (Mead Johnson) chemotherapy.

******

575. **EPILEPTICS:** Most epileptic patients have an urinary pH of 8 or 9. Reducing pH to normal reduces severity and frequency of epilepsy.

******

576. **DEXTROAMPHETAMINE HELPFUL IN EPILEPTIC PATIENTS:** It combats drowsiness induced by anticonvulsants and it is sometimes effective alone in certain types of focal epilepsy. It appears to be the most effective agent in combating sleep seizures.

******

577. **INCREASES PHOSPHATE POISONING:** When treating organic phosphate poisoning, avoid opiates, aminophyline, tranquilizers, and Lasix® (National) in the treatment. They add to the toxicity.

******

578. **DO NOT** use Liquamycin® (Pfizer) in small animals, particularly intramuscular.

******

579. **DOGS REQUIRE MORE THYROID:** Dogs tolerate 28 times more desiccated thyroid than people. A sign of over-dosing in dogs is sneezing. Reduction of dose eliminates the sneezing. A twenty pound Dachshund will tolerate and respond well to 5 grains of fresh dessicated thyroid.

******

580. **RESPONSE IMPORTANT:** Response to thyroid therapy is the best method of diagnosis for a practitioner. Three to six weeks are needed to get response.

******

581. **I.V. POTASSIUM PENICILLIN LETHAL:** Don't use potassium penicillin intravenously in dogs or cats. Potassium may cause cardiac irregularities and even cardiac arrest if given rapidly.

582. **SYMPTOMS OF ORGANIC PHOSPHATE POISONING:**
   A. Depression.
   B. Salivation.
   C. Rapid respiration.
   D. Muscle tremors (more severe cases may have wobbly gait or semi-paralysis).
   E. Hyper-peristalsis with diarrhea.
   F. Coma or convulsions prior to death.

The following animals are listed in order of their susceptibility to organic phosphate poisoning: cat, sheep, dog, horse, cow.

For the treatment of organic phosphate poisoning in severe cases, give atropine intravenously at the rate of 1 mg./10 lbs. repeated as often as 15 minutes to 4 hours. In less severe cases, the same dose can be used at 4 to 8 hour intervals. Atropine therapy should be repeated for 24 to 36 hours. Within a few minutes after atropine therapy, there should be a cessation of muscle tremors and dilation of the pupils. If this does not occur, additional atropine should be considered. Usually there is a rapid recovery in the animal treated early after exposure. Cats have been noted to have tremors for several days after exposure. These tremors disappear each time atropine is given.

* * * * * *

583. **AVOID** giving chloramphenicol with belladonna, phenobarbitol, or tranquilizers.

* * * * * *

584. **TSH DEFICIENCY:** Acanthosis nigricans is thought to be a TSH (thyroid stimulating hormone) deficiency (dermatropic fraction) with secondary hypothyroidism and hypocorticism. Cases exhibit severe otitis, bacterial and fungal infections of the skin. They often relapse. In beginning the case, give TSH 5 days and Propycil® (Jensen-Salsbery) for 21 days. If caught early, it may not relapse. The Prednameen® (Summit Hill) or Bucoderm® (Burns-Biotec) type oral products can be massaged in topically and seem beneficial in 20 ml. solution add 2 ml. Combiotic® (Pfizer) and 100 mg. neomycin. Sex hormones and low level steroids may help. DMSO in 40-6-% solution with steroids topically is sometimes dramatic in scleraderma.

* * * * * *

585. **IN CASES OF SERTOLI CELL TUMOR,** the nipples enlarge from the front to the back. In gonadal adrenal dysfunction, the reverse may be true. The nipples often stay enlarged if condition is corrected.

586. **HIVES:** Boxers and Boston Terriers urticate easily. They have a larger number of mast cells in their skin. One-fourth cc. 1:1000 Adrenalin® (Parke-Davis) is the best treatment. Administer antihistamines intravenously only. Steroids subcutaneous or intramuscular are of little value.

* * * * * *

587. **DRY EYES:** For a better diagnosis and more accurate prognosis in cases of keratoconjunctivitis sicca, use a Schirmer Teat Test Strip® (Tilden Yates). Leave the strip in the eye for 1 minute. Interpret as follows: normal = more than 15 mm.; suspect = 9 mm. to 15 mm.; positive keratoconjunctivitis sicca = less than 9 mm.

* * * * * *

588. **NASOLACRIMAL PATENCY:** Passage of fluorescein from the eye to the external nares is a reasonable test for patency of the nasolacrimal system. A strip of fluorescein is applied to the upper bulbar conjunctiva and moistened with two drops of 0.5% methylcellulose, Isopto® plain, (Alcon). The dye usually appears at the external nares in 3 to 5 minutes. Both sides should be performed at the same time to compare passage times. Ultraviolet light enhances detection of the dye in cats.

* * * * * *

589. **UNRELIABLE:** Fluorescein passage in brachiocephalic dogs is not reliable. The dye may exist more readily in the nasopharynx. The dog's tongue and saliva should be examined with the Wood's Lamp.

* * * * * *

590. **WOOD'S LAMP:** After fluorescein has been instilled in an animal's eye, examination with a Wood's Lamp makes even the smallest scratch or foreign body show up vividly.

* * * * * *

591. **USE A BLUE LIGHT:** Corneal abrasions are usually diagnosed after the cornea has been stained with fluorescein. Abrasions stand out clearly if a blue light, rather than the standard white flashlight, is used for illumination.

* * * * * *

592. **INEXPENSIVE LIGHT:** Blue penlights are commercially available and relatively expensive. Blue cellophane or crepe paper held over the flashlight with an elastic band works just as well. In a pinch, the green light on every ophthalmoscope is better than a white light, but not as good as the blue light.

* * * * * *

593. **SUPERIOR STAIN:** Rose bengal is used infrequently in veterinary medicine, although it is a valuable stain in the evaluation of health of the corneal and conjunctival epithelium. A vital stain, rose bengal stains dead and degenerating epithelium and mucus a brilliant red. Rose bengal is retained excessively by the cornea and conjunctiva in canine and feline keratoconjunctivitis sicca, pigmentary keratitis, exposure keratitis, and certain corneal ulcers.

******

594. **EYE HEALING OIL (CASTOR OIL):** Prepare it in ¼ oz. dropper bottles and instruct clients to use it in their pet's eyes prior to bathing or to protect hunting dogs before sending them through brush and weeds. We charge 50 cents per ¼ oz. to cover the medicine and the "conversation" that goes along with dispensing.

******

595. **KEEP GLOBE MOIST:** When a dog is to be brought in with a prolapsed eye, advise the client to keep the globe moist with maple or Karo® syrup (not vaseline) until the animal arrives at the hospital.

******

596. **CONTACT LENS SOLUTION:** Adapt® solution (contact lens solution) is recommended by many for keratitis sicca (dry eyes) and it can be mixed with Anaprime® (Diamond) or Gentocin® (Schering) drops for standard eye treatments. This solution persists in the eye for 4-6 hours.

******

597. **EDTA HELPFUL IN ULCERS:** Sequesterol®, EDTA, 12-15 drops in 15 ml. For eye ulcers administer one drop per minute for six minutes, four times a day.

******

598. **TAPE DEWCLAWS:** When treating an eye condition associated with any pruritus in the dog, tape the dewclaws on the front feet to prevent self-inflicted trauma.

******

599. **GLUE EYELIDS:** When a conjunctival flap is needed in the treatment of corneal ulcers, glue the lids together with 1 - 2 drops of Super Glue®.

******

600. **PROGRESSIVE EXOPHTHALOMES** is usually caused by a retrobulbar tumor.

******

601. AN EYE WASH PREPARATION WHICH CAN BE PREPARED BY THE GALLON.

½ oz. bicarbonate of soda (baking soda)

½ oz. boric acid, USP

½ oz. table salt

2 oz. glycerin, USP

4 cc. of 10% concentrated Roccal® (Winthrop).

To make a 10% Roccal® solution use 26 oz. of the 50% concentrated Roccal® in one gallon of water. Use only 4 cc. of this dilute mixture to one gallon of eye wash to make a 1-10,000 dilution. Use the 10% Roccal® solution for hypodermic syringes, cleansing of table tops between examination, etc. by diluting it in a proportion of 1½ to 2 oz. of the 10% solution in one gallon of water. The 10% Roccal® used for eye wash can be taken from the gallon mixture with a 5 cc., hypodermic syringe to the 4 cc. mark. Measure carefully. The eye wash is prepared as follows: Put ½ oz. of boric acid into a clean gallon jar. Add hot tap water to fill ¼ to ½ of the gallon. Then add baking soda and shake well until disolved. Add salt, glycerin, and Roccal® and fill the jar, slowly, with tap water to make a full gallon.

******

602. GARLIC HELPFUL:
An aid in the treatment of acute bronchitis and other upper respiratory inflammations in dogs and cats is oil of garlic given in gelatin capsules. The capsules can be obtained from mail-order suppliers and nutrition stores. Vary the dose from one to two capsules t.i.d. or q.i.d. or even hourly, depending on the size of the patient and the severity of the condition. In many cases of acute bronchitis where this treatment has been used as the sole therapeutic agent, coughing ceases or is greatly relieved within 24 hours.

******

603. PULMONARY SOUNDS AID DIAGNOSIS:
When a dog is doing more wheezing than coughing, suspect a collapsed or partially occluded trachea distal to the bifurcation.

Ronchi are heard on exhalation. They are usually dry, while rales are heard on inspiration and vary in moistness.

In dogs with pulmonary fibrosis, the bronchovesicular sounds are dry, interrupted, creaky and extend throughout inspiration and expiration. They are produced by extension and retraction of the fibrous tissue. If they are bilateral, they may produce accentuation of the second heart sound, and cor pulmonale.

Extensive, long standing bronchopneumonia may produce bronchiectesis, hypertension, and right-side cardiac failure. So called emphysematous crackling sounds are heard on auscultation, accompanied by sclerotic rales and ronchi. Usually no cardiac murmurs are heard and the white blood cell count is elevated.

* * * * * *

604. **NONCARDIAC COUGH:** Script or order Isuprel® (Winthrop) for noncardiac coughs. Give 1-2 ml/10lbs., t.i.d..

* * * * * *

605. **REVERSE SNEEZE** is a reflex like cough originating in the nasal mucosa, by a rapid, deep, inspiration, often with the head held parallel to the floor.

* * * * * *

606. **GERIATRIC MEDICATION:** If you encounter a heart beat in a resting dog of 160 or more, think of digitilization. Old dogs need four times as much thiamine as do young dogs. Also, vitamins C and E may help geriatric patients. Try using Metrazol® (Summit Hill) , 1 tablet b.i.d., for incontinence in old male dogs. If chronic cystitis does not respond to antibiotics alone, try steroids with antibiotics. You may be dealing with an allergy.

* * * * * *

607. **OLIVE OIL AND BAY RUM:** A good combination for keeping a dog's coat and skin soft and oily, is equal parts of olive oil and bay rum. To apply, a small amount of the mixture is rubbed into the coat. The treatment is not recommended for poodles.

* * * * * *

608. **HOT SPOT THERAPY:** A treatment for acute moist dermatitis: 1 lb. tannic acid N.F. powder, 1 lb. salacylic acid USP (fine crystals), and isopropyl alcohol QS to make 5 gallons. Instruct the client to pour the solution on the moist lesion and scrub the site with a toothbrush once or twice daily (depending on the severity of the condition) for 3 - 4 days. The scrubbing facilitates penetration of the solution and removal of scabs. Many "hot spots" dry up quickly with this treatment.

* * * * * *

609. **FERRIC SUBSULFATE:** Moist dermatitis (hot spots) clear up quickly when treated with ferric subsulfate solution applied once a day. The treatment should be used in conjunction with an injection of cortisone

and penicillin-strepomycin.

* * * * * *

610. **HASTENS HEALING:** A skin cream was developed years ago for baby eczema. It is very soothing and hastens granulation and the healing of the acute moist dermatitis lesions. The ingredients are as follows:

    10 ounce of zinc oxide, USP
    1 ounce of benzocaine powder, USP
    5 pounds of cold cream, USP

This is an excellent preparation for dry eczema areas; to heal acute moist dermatitis lesions after they are "dry"; for dry, irritated elbows on the large breeds of dogs; and for irritated anal areas.

* * * * * *

611. **ZINC WILL IMPROVE THE HAIR COAT** in most animals and reduce hyperkeratosis associated with a deficiency syndrome.

* * * * * *

612. **CALCIUM THERAPY** is a must in old dogs with skin and kidney lesions. It is often overlooked in cases where there is allergy and inflammation.

* * * * * *

613. **IMPROVE IMMUNITY:** When you encounter a chronic skin condition, try treatment with calcium pantothenate. A deficiency of calcium pantothenate is reported to reduce an animal's ability to produce antibodies.

* * * * * *

614. **REDUCE SHEDDING:** For shedding hair problems in the normal looking short haired dog use 8 oz. glycerine, 8 oz. water, 1 tablespoon vinegar. Rub down daily. 1 oz. of Roccal® (Winthrop) can be added if mild dermatitis is present.

* * * * * *

615. **COLLIE NOSE:** Treat by painting daily with zinc oxide or Pellitol™ (Pitman Moore).

* * * * * *

616. **D.N.P.® FOR WARTS:** When many warts appear suddenly in the mouth they will often drop off in four days after 1 cc./10 lb. D.N.P.® (American Cyanamide) is administered. This therapy is not effective if the warts have been present for some time or appeared slowly.

* * * * * *

617. **HORNY GROWTHS** on the nose may respond to vitamin A injections

and castor oil topically, or 10% salicyclic acid. Horny pads may have to be removed surgically.

******

618. **INTERDIGITAL CYST:** Administer 1 mg. of 1-throxine sodium for 3 weeks. If there is no response, put on Terramycin® for 1 week with Vetalog® (Squibb) and then continue Vetalog® (Pfizer) tablets every other morning (dose to effect) forever, if needed.

******

619. **MEDICATED SHAMPOO:** When treating fungus skin infections with shampoos, allow them to remain in contact with the skin for several hours.

******

620. **FLEA ALLERGY** is a delayed allergy (seven days after bite) so don't be fooled if the owner has bathed the dog in Skip Flea Soap® before the office visit. If fleas are scarce, spray or powder well.

******

621. **ATOPY:** Wirehair Fox Terriers and Dalmations have a higher incidence of hay fever (Atopy), starting at age 2-3 years. They rub eyes, scratch face on rug, lick feet, and scratch ears and axilla. Atopy is seasonal with ragweed from August through December, or all year with house dust. Some don't scratch, just cough. Skin test may not be positive except at the end of the season. Provocative test for house dust: Place dog in enclosed shower and shake rug (get out of shower).

******

622. **DISTILLED WATER** should be used in preparing special diets for animals with suspected food allergies because of molds and chemicals in public water supplies.

******

623. **NEUTO-DERMATITIS OF SIAMESE CATS:** Amputation of the tail is useless. Tranquilizers, phenobarbital, and Dilantin® (Pakre-Davis) are usually transient or of no benefit. Most cases respond quickly to primidone, Mysoline® (Ayerst) half a 50 mg. tablet b.i.d.. Medication can be gradually reduced or discontinued depending on the cat's response.

******

624. **LONG TERM ANTIBIOTICS:** Paronychia, an inflammation of the nail fold, is usually bacterial in origin and frequently complicated by

licking and trauma. Surface cultures are difficult to evaluate; consequently, punch biopsy may yield more valid results. Treatment should be directed toward elimination of the cause and relief of the frequently intense pruritis. Appropriate long term antibiotic therapy combined with daily soaking and bandaging with a soothing ointment such as Pellitol™ (Pitman-Moore) are necessary.

******

625. **VITAMINS HELPFUL IN SKIN DISEASE:** Vitamin C may help pyodermas; vitamin A may help fungal diseases and follicular diseases. Vitamins E and D won't hurt. Vitamin E and selenium have benefited a few chronic skin cases. Panothenic acid is concerned with pigmentation of hair and skin.

******

626. **ANAL GLANDS** may be a source of bacteria or contribute to bacterial allergic syndromes. Anal glands often respond to flushing with detergent and instilling 5% sodium morrhuate. Another method is to flush and instill with V-Tergent 8X™ (Pitman-Moore). Leave it in.

******

627. **ADOLPH'S MEAT TENDERIZER:** Large ulcerated and traumatized areas of skin infection sometimes clear up more quickly if they are treated with Adolph's Meat Tenderizer®.

******

628. **SARAN WRAP®:** Old wounds that are severly edematous can often be successfully sutured after being sweated under a Furacin® (Norden) pack covered with plastic wrap (Saran Wrap®). Sweat for ten or twelve hours followed by thorough debridement. A systemic diuretic will also aid in reducing swelling in these wounds.

******

629. **WOUND THERAPY FOR NON-SUTURABLE AREAS:** Add Dermafur® plus insulin to a vitamin A capsule and mix well. (Small amount of insulin, ¼ cc., is all that is needed.)

******

630. **LICK GRANULOMA:** Give Nyloxin® (Hynson, Westcott, Dunning -cobra venom) to control this problem. One cc. weekly, subcutaneously, for 3 to 5 weeks. It is also useful for other pain problems such as osteo-arthritic pain and disc pain.

******

631. **ICE REMOVES GUM:** To remove chewing gum or a small spot of tar, hold a piece of ice on area to harden the material.

******

632. **SEBORRHEA ITCHY:** Seborrhic dermatitis is itchy. Pragmatar® (Norden) shampoo and/or ointment is usually the treatment of choice topically. If these don't work, switch. Sulfur, onions, carrots, and raw liver in the diet helps.

******

633. **REDUCE SCALING:** As an aid in reducing scaling and controlling seborrhea, add 2 - 4 cc. of Vetalog® (Squibb) to medicated shampoos. Allow the shampoo to soak on the dog for 15 minutes or more and then rinse with creme rinse. The treatment should be repeated whenever scaling begins to appear.

******

634. **OIL TREATMENT FOR DRY SKIN:** Too many medicated baths dry a dog's skin. Alternate with Sardo® or Alpha Keri® .

******

635. **SOAPLESS CLEANING:** In the treatment of seborrhea, cleansing the skin is very important. DO NOT bath with soaps, shampoos, or detergents unless absolutely necessary. Use a 1:20 mixture of bath oil and water (*i.e.*, Alpha Keri®) and cleanse and moisturize the skin daily. This can be accomplished by bathing or spot treatment with a bottle and sprayer. This form of "soapless cleansing" is excellent for disordered skin. It is gentle and effective. The water softens and dissolves dirt while some soaks into the skin to moisturize it. Seborrhea means that the skin oils are being produced to excess and/or that these oils do not contain the normal oils and waxes necessary for healthy skin.

******

636. **TREATMENT FOR SARCOPTIC MANGE IN THE DOG:** Prescribe thiabendazole, Mintezol® (Merck). The Mintezol® should be given orally and applied topically twice daily for one week. In addition, an insecticidal shampoo or dip should be used weekly over the entire body of the dog to help control the condition.

******

637. **TOPICAL RONNEL:** It is irritating to both the dog's skin and human skin. Anyone applying this compound should wear rubber gloves. Also, great care must be exerted to see that the mixture is formulated properly as

well as mixed thoroughly. One veterinary school reported two deaths from the use of this mixture, but that may have been due to improper mixing. The formula must be agitated throughly each time before use. Caution the owners about its possible toxicity to both dogs and humans.

SCOTT'S FORMULA (7.7% ronnel)
365 ml. ronnel concentrate, Ectoral™ (Pitman Moore)
900 ml. propylene glycol
150 ml. isopropyl alcohol
Rub mixture in well to 1/3 dog's body a day.

WEAR RUBBER GLOVES!

******

638. **REMOVAL OF ASCITIC FLUID** is likely to cause collapse if the animal is on a low sodium diet.

******

639. **OLD CARDIAC PATIENTS:** Routinely use Canalb™ (Pitman-Moore) protein solution in the old cardiac patient during surgical procedures. Using an intravenous drip, a slow continuous administration of Canalb™ insures adequate blood pressure and it may help prevent pulmonary edema or ascites that may accompany salt solutions.

******

640. **REPLACE POTASSIUM:** Dogs lose three times as much potassium in vomiting. In CHF (congestive heart failure) associated with uremia and vomiting try to gently replace potassium. Potassium loss will produce unusual behavioral changes and poor appetite. Sodium loss decreases activity and response.

******

641. **DISTILLED WATER:** Animals with congestive heart failure should be offered distilled water. Many water supplies are softened and contain high sodium levels.

******

642. **COCKER SPANIEL MALES** have three times as much congestive heart failure as other males, and six times as much as Cocker females.

******

643. **HORMONES HELP HEART:** Dr. W. Stumpf, University of North Carolina, has found that a portion of the heart reacts to estradiol; strengthening the hypothesis that female sex hormones guard women against heart disease.

HEART RATES

644. **HEART RATE IS FAST** in excitement, shock, after some drugs, anemia, congestive heart failure, fever, severe hemorrhage, myocarditis.

* * * * * *

645. **HEART RATE IS SLOW** in brain tumors or increased intracranial pressure, with jaundice malnutrition, thyroidial imbalances.

* * * * * *

646. **HEART RATE IS FAST** in heart conditions such as nodal tachycardia, atrial tachycardia, atrial flutter with 2:1 block, paroxysmal ventricular tachycardia.

* * * * * *

647. **HEART RATE IS SLOW** in heart conditions such a.v. nodal rhythm, complete a.v. block, incomplete A.V. block with dropped beats, S.A. block. Also, normally slower in sinus arrhythmia than when exercised.

* * * * * *

648. **IN GENERAL,** heart rates on initial table examination are not diagnostic of any heart disease.

COMMON ERRORS

649. **IT IS AN ERROR** to use stock fluoroscein solutions for corneal staining.

* * * * * *

650. **IT IS AN ERROR** to assume:
  A. If pupil responds to light — vision present.
  B. If pupil does not respond to light — vision gone.

* * * * * *

651. **ANTIBIOTICS ARE COMMONLY MISUSED.** If continued too long the condition remains stagnant.

* * * * * *

652. **IT IS A MISTAKE** to continue using steroids where contraindicated (ulceration) or useless.

* * * * * *

653. **IT IS WRONG** to use topical anesthetics alone or in combination for treatment purposes.

* * * * * *

654. **EPISCLERITIS** — often diagnosed as tumor or hyperplasia. It is an allergic manifestation. Responds dramatically to steroids (subconjunctival injection).

******

655. **CONJUNCTIVA** — hypertrophy of membrane nictitans often mistaken for eversion of the membrane nictitans (and vice-versa). **Do not** remove the structure for either condition.
Hypertrophy - treat medically (steroids).
Eversion - treat surgically

******

656. **PURULENT CONJUNCTIVITIS.** It is an error to assume every case of conjuctival discharge is a primary conjunctivitis - especially if unilateral.

******

657. **KERATOCONJUNCTIVITIS SICCA.** The failure to recognize is the most frequent error in diagnosis concerning the conjunctiva and cornea. Sticky, stringy discharge. Red, thickened, velvety conjunctiva. Corneal pathology, light stain, dull dry appearance. Discomfort (squinting). Possible dry nostril.

******

658. **PIGMENTARY KERATITIS.** It is an error to assume it is a primary disease entity. Causes:
   A. Stress (distichiasis, nasal folds, entropion, conjunctivitis, keratitis sicca, pannus).
   B. Following and accompanying superficial vascularization.
   C. Sequela to interstitial keratitis.
   D. Migration of uveal pigment following prolapse.
Treatment: eliminate cause before being concerned with pigment.

******

659. **DEEP ULCERATION.** It is wrong to assume good healing is in progress if a "clear" area is present. It could be exposed descemet's membrane. Treatment: conjunctival flap.

******

660. **IRITIS.** A common error is to diagnose as something else. Failure to recognize and institute proper treatment results in serious complications. Treatment: Atropine, steroids (subconjunctival). Do not depend on topical anesthesia (*e.g.* tetracaine) for pain relief. Atropine is preferable.

******

661. **GLAUCOMA.** Often it is not recognized in its acute congestive phase and proper treatment is not started immediately.

******

662. **IT IS AN ERROR** to diagnose cataract when nuclear sclerosis is responsible for loss of translucency.

******

663. **CATARACT** can be secondary to progressive retinal atrophy. To suggest surgery is in error.

******

664. **ORBIT** — common error is to diagnose exophthalmos as glaucoma.

******

665. **ANTIBIOTICS** (e.g., penicillin) used systemically for intra-ocular infection are useless. Must know which antibiotic can penetrate the blood-aqueous barrier. Chloramphenicol does.

EXOTICS

666. **AVIAN/SMALL MAMMAL EXAMINATION AND LIGHT SURGICAL PROCEDURE DOSAGE:** Ketamine Dosage intramuscularly or subcutaneously. Canaries — 1 mg.; Parakeets — 2 mg.; small Parrots, Love Birds, Guinea Pigs, Hamsters, Gerbils, Mice — 5 mg.; Squirrels, large Parrots, Rats — 10 mg.; small Monkeys, Ferrets, Skunks, Raccoons, Kinkajou — 15-20 mg. Dosage may be increased, if necessary, for surgical anesthesia by 1.5 or 2X.

******

667. **LIGHTS OFF:** Pet birds can be removed from cages for examination with minimal restraint if the room lights are turned off first.

****

668. **SICK BIRDS** are always cold and require heat. You can maintain a cage temperature of 80-85⁰ F. by placing the cage on a heating pad and wrapping the sides, top and back, with clear plastic wrap. Cover only two-thirds to three-fourths of the front of the cage to allow adequate ventilation. Place a thermometer inside; if the temperature goes too high, put newspapers or towels between the cage and heating pad. The amount of plastic wrap can be varied as long as the cage is not airtight. The clear plastic wrap allows maintenance of normal photo periods, encouraging birds to eat normally.

******

669. **MALNUTRITION:** Many caged birds suffer malnutrition because of poor eating habits. No attempt should be made to starve a bird into eating new foods. A small bird can die within 48 hours if it doesn't eat. Methods to improve a bird's eating habits include:

    A. Sweeten the water. Later add other nutrients such as juices, milk, and Neo-Mullsoy® (Syntex). Neo-Mullsoy® is a liquid soy protein that can be obtained at any pharmacy without prescription.

    B. Introduce only small amounts of new food.

    C. Feed hot foods such as hot nuts, cereals, cheese, and soup.

    D. Mix new foods with the routine basic feed.

    E. Place new foods below a mirror or next to a favorite toy.

    F. Try feeding outside the cage.

    G. Change feeding from *ad libitum* to three 15-minute feeding periods.

    H. Hand or spoon feed.

******

670. **SCIENCE DIET® FOR MYNAHS:** Some mynah birds and parrots do very well on Science Diet® (Hills) soft billed bird food.

******

671. **ENTERITIS THERAPY:** When a serious outbreak of enteritis occurs in a parakeet or canary aviary, giving the antidiarrheal agent Biosol-M® (Upjohn) is a effective way of buying time until a diagnosis can be established. Dispense 10 c.c. of Biosol-M® in 2 oz. of lixotinic, or VAL Syrup® (Fort Dodge) and prescribe a dose of 2 to 4 drops in each ounce of drinking water. In severe outbreaks, the dosage can be increased to 10 drops/1 oz. water. If the diarrhea persists or recurs while the birds are still being given the antidiarrheal agent; chloromycetin, ampicillin, or nitrofurazone can be added to the Biosol-M® mixture. The birds can be induced to drink more of the medicated water if the temperature in the aviary is raised to 85° F.

******

672. **HYPERTROPHY OF THE THYROID GLAND** causes severe respiratory problems in parakeets. All parakeets need iodine therapy throughout their lives. Many birds are treated for pneumonia or respiratory tract infections, when actually they have only respiratory embarrassment from enlargement of the thyroid gland. Add small amount of iodine to drinking water.

******

673. **FEVERISH BIRDS NEED SUGAR:** Birds showing whitish diarrhea usually also have a fever. The feverish bird loses flesh more rapidly because it burns proteins to produce calories. This results in high elimination of urates with resulting white diarrhea. It is necessary to supply sugar and honey as a food supplement. If the bird does not eat, give the sugar in the drinking water because the bird will continue to drink as a consequence of the fever.

* * * * * *

674. **EXCESS FAT:** Parakeets often suffer from the hepatitis-enteritis syndrome. They go light, become anemic, and develop diarrhea and reddish abdomen. The cause is excess of fats in diets (rich seeds). They develop fatty livers and sometimes lipomas. Treat with Biosol-M® (Upjohn) and lixotinic preparation (liver supplement, choline, and B-vitamins) and change diet to only millet and groats. Keep warm and avoid further stress.

* * * * * *

675. **IN PROLONGED MOULT,** always include sulfur containing amino acids in the therapy. This can be accomplished by adding greens such as cabbage and onions. These vegetables contain the needed methionine for good feather formation.

* * * * * *

676. **FLUSH SINUSES:** Parrots often suffer from infectious sinusitis characterized by clogged nostrils or purulent discharge. Treatment is to remove debris with a toothpick and flush medication directly into nostrils. Use a combination of saline, DMSO, chloramphenicol and Tylocine® (Elanco). (5 cc. saline, ½ cc. DMSO, ½ cc. chloramphenicol and ½ cc. Tylocine®). Flush 2-3 drops t.i.d.. Add vitamins to water, especially vitamin A.

* * * * * *

677. **CEREBRAL HEMORRHAGE:** If a usually healthy bird dies within 48 hours or less, always check for the possibility of cerebral hemorrhage. It is necessary to skin the skull. The blood clot becomes visible through the exposed bone.

* * * * * *

CONTRIBUTOR'S INDEX

A.

Anderson, D., DVM, 523

Antelyes, J., DVM, 107

Austin, V.H., DVM, 137

B.

Baker, E., DVM, 14, 133

Baker, J.R., DVM, 291

Barkham, T.W., DVM, 65

Barnett, R.E., DVM, 207

Barrett, R.B., DVM, 109

Barry, A.A., DVM, 162, 377

Beeman, M., DVM, 493

Bellhorn, T., DVM, 265

Berg, P., DVM, 208

Bernstein, K., DVM, 426

Berryhill, G., DVM, 108, 173, 385

Bild, C., DVM, 187, 248, 251, 384, 469

Blakemore, J., DVM, 422

Boam, G.W., DVM, 267

Bone, W.J., DVM, 378

Brasmer, T., DVM, 157

Brinker, W., DVM, 268

Brooks, C., DVM, 112

Brown, R., DVM, 278

Brumble, G., DVM, 209

Brutus, R.L., DVM, 172

Burch, G., DVM, 1, 2, 3, 4, 5, 6, 7, 8, 9, 10, 22, 23, 25, 27, 40,42, 43, 51, 52, 55, 73, 77, 78, 79, 84, 90, 91, 92, 93, 94, 121, 184, 215, 301, 310, 363, 420, 482,

C.

Carbone, M.G., DVM, 257

Casler, B., DVM, 60

Clarke, R.P., DVM, 118

Cockrell, K., DVM, 375

Cohen, R.H., DVM, 120

Collins, J.R., DVM, 122

Cook, C.L., DVM, 48

Cooper, H.K., DVM, 394

Cohen, A., DVM, 154

Crago, V.G., DVM, 171

Crane, S.W., DVM, 255, 304

Cutter, A., DVM, 386

D.

Davidson, J.L., DVM, 538

Dee, J., DVM, 163

Dehne, G.W., DVM, 75, 110, 376

Dingel, R.M., DVM, 233

Doering, G., DVM, 393, 458, 566

Dolphin, R.E., DVM, 569

Donohue, B.T., DVM, 277

Dwelle, E.D., DVM, 66

E.

Eckert, R.R., DVM, 174

Ehrenzweig, J., DVM, 452

Ellyn, G., DVM, 289

Emerson, B., DVM, 274

Ernest, D.M., DVM, 442, 454

F.

Fallon, H.J., DVM, 19, 159, 337, 399

Fish, R.W., DVM, 415

Fishler, J.J., DVM, 357, 410

Fiske, R.A., DVM, 369

Fincher, D.S., DVM, 333

Fletcher, K.C., DVM, 217

Foley, R.J., DVM, 67

Fox, L.M., DVM, 72

Fowler, V.W., DVM, 175

Frey, D.C., DVM, 105, 505

Fridya, L.M., DVM, 282

Fuller, W.J., DVM, 242, 409

G.

Gaines Dog Progress Digest, 485

Garcia, E., DVM, 225, 499, 567

Gilbert, A.H., DVM, 380

Givens, P.M., DVM, 181, 498

Glasofer, S., DVM, 16, 17, 20, 26, 28, 29, 30, 31, 32, 33, 35, 50, 54, 56, 59, 74, 191, 195, 196, 197, 199, 200, 202, 206, 210, 212, 214, 218, 226, 228, 232, 237, 240, 245, 259, 269, 273, 275, 286, 287, 332, 450, 488, 489, 493, 496, 497, 513, 533

Gomez, C., DVM, 220

Gray, J.J., DVM, 147

Gross, J., 223, 263, 494

H.

Hall, C.G., DVM, 265, 552

Halliwell, R., DVM, 346

Hansen, A.G., DVM, 252

Hansen, J.S., DVM, 398

Hawaii (Univ. of)—Vet Digest, 484

Haynes, B., 365

Holtzman, J., DVM, 431

Hogg, A., DVM, 249

Hopper, J.E., DVM, 122

Hoskins, J., DVM, 123

Hugenbert, J., DVM, 448

Hyatt, R., DVM, 190

I.

Iowa State Univ. Newsletter, 331, 389

J.

Jackson, W.F., 11, 12, 14, 15, 24, 111, 114, 126, 186, 221, 222, 224, 237, 285, 295, 308, 368, 463, 464, 465, 487, 527, 529, 544, 545, 554, 565, 578, 584, 586, 597, 603, 604, 605, 614, 616, 618, 621, 626, 627, 632, 638, 640, 642

Johnston, D.E., DVM, 321

Jolley, W., DVM, 571

Jones, A.O., DVM, 165, 256, 542

Jones, R.G., DVM, 503

K.

Katsinis, N.D., DVM, 532

Kavit, A.Y., DVM, 161, 447, 453, 525

Keller, W.F., DVM, 411, 412

Kelly, H.W., DVM, 241, 470

Kelley, W.C., DVM, 209

King, J., DVM, 366

Kipnis, R., DVM, 64, 115

Klaudt, J.J., DVM, 204, 480

Knecht, C.D., DVM, 258, 347

Knowles, R., DVM, 129

Knox, D.W., 382

Koch, S.A., VMD, 413, 595

Kretz, W.H., MD, 262

L.

Landis, P., VMD, 144, 336, 536

Leach, D., DVM, 353

Lefeber, T.J., DVM, 669

Lemmon, M.W., 602

Levinson, F., DVM, 271, 507

Levoy, R.P., 39, 41, 44, 45, 46, 62, 76, 81, 82, 83, 85, 86, 87, 88, 89

Lewis, H.T., DVM, 183, 471

Lorenz, M.D., DVM, 345

M.

Mabry, A.J., DVM, 178

Magrane, H., DVM, 472, 594, 601, 610

Magrane, W., DVM, 649, 650, 651, 652, 653, 654, 655, 656, 657, 658, 659, 660, 661, 662, 663, 664

Mandelker, L., DVM, 21, 58, 117, 136, 151, 152, 155, 168, 170, 172, 180, 227, 234, 235, 236, 238, 261, 270, 280, 281, 296, 299, 306, 312, 313, 316, 317, 319, 320, 322, 323, 361, 372, 381, 387, 404, 427, 443, 459, 477, 495, 501, 515, 534, 535, 555, 557, 561, 570, 572, 574, 576, 581, 629, 633, 636, 639, 666, 671, 673, 674, 675, 676, 677

Meagee, H., DVM, 606

McMichael, D.A., DVM, 516

McNicol, W.E., DVM, 63, 513

Medical World News, 350

Merry, L.M., DVM, 260

Meyer, B.A., DVM, 229

Morrill, W.E., DVM, 205

Mosier, J.E., DVM, 284, 300, 330, 539

N.

Nebraska Extension Newsletter, 445

Nelms, J.W., VMD, 34, 71

O.

Oeheme, F., DVM, 550

Oregon Animal Health News, 326

Osborne, C., DVM, 440

Ott, R.L., DVM, 139. 140

P.

Pedersen, N.C., DVM, 425

Pennsylvania State Univ., 294

Phillips, G., DVM, 272
Place, M., DVM, 376
Purvis, J.P., DVM, 609

Spencer, J., DVM, 519
Stauffer, V.D., DVM, 446
Stolfus, T.A., DVM, 211
Stried, R.O., DVM, 167

R.

Ray, J.R., DVM, 69, 168, 182, 335, 392, 468, 521
Reeves, K.F., DVM, 590
Riley, M.D., DVM, 508
Robbins, G., DVM, 559
Roberts, K., DVM, 274
Rousseau, J., DVM, 219

T.

Tayman, D., DVM, 37, 164, 198, 246, 279, 383, 413, 473, 474, 512
Thomas, R.D., DVM, 449
Thompson, E.E., DVM, 150
Tiekert, C.G., DVM, 414
Timm, O.H., 283
Turner, M.E., DVM, 490
Turrou, R.M., DVM, 156

S.

Salsbury, D.L., DVM, 401, 456
Samuelson, M.L., DVM, 423
Schenk, C.T., DVM, 13
Schmidt, G., DVM, 587
Schobert, T. DVM, 448
Schumacher, H., DVM, 177, 201, 266, 479, 509, 514, 537
Schwartzman, I.W., DVM, 53, 213
Schwartzman, R.M., DVM, 344
Schwichtenberg, A.E., DVM, 220
Scott, D.W., DVM, 531
Scott, W.W., DVM, 637
Sherman, L.A., DVM, 122, 276
Shulak, F.B., DVM, 124
Smith, E., DVM, 457

V.

Vanderhof, R., DVM, 492
Vankruiningen, H., DVM, 563

W.

Wagner, A., DVM, 568
Wallace, L.J., DVM, 481
Watkins, J.B., DVM, 510
Webb, W.G., DVM, 371
Whitney, W.H., DVM, 95
Wittig, J., DVM, 405
Wysong, R.L., DVM, 179, 209, 254, 370, 373, 506